# Legal Issues and Ethical Dilemmas in Respiratory Care

# Legal Issues and Ethical Dilemmas in Respiratory Care

Charles Carroll, EdD, RRT
Dean
Division of Health Careers and Wellness
Formerly, Professor and Program Director
Respiratory Care Program
Daytona Beach Community College
Daytona Beach, Florida

F. A. DAVIS COMPANY • Philadelphia

F. A. Davis Company
1915 Arch Street
Philadelphia, PA 19103

Copyright © 1996 by F. A. Davis Company

All rights reserved. This book is protected by copyright. No part of it may be reproduced, stored in a retrieval system, or transmitted in any form or by any means, electronic, mechanical, photocopying, recording, or otherwise, without written permission from the publisher.

Printed in the United States of America

Last digit indicates print number: 10 9 8 7 6 5 4 3 2 1

*Publisher, Allied Health:* Jean-François Vilain
*Acquisitions Editor:* Lynn Borders Caldwell
*Developmental Editor:* Crystal McNichol
*Production Editor:* Glenn L. Fechner
*Cover Designer:* Louis J. Forgione

As new scientific information becomes available through basic and clinical research, recommended treatments and drug therapies undergo changes. The author and publisher have done everything possible to make this book accurate, up to date, and in accord with accepted standards at the time of publication. The author, editors, and publisher are not responsible for errors or omissions or for consequences from application of the book, and make no warranty, expressed or implied, in regard to the contents of the book. Any practice described in this book should be applied by the reader in accordance with professional standards of care used in regard to the unique circumstances that may apply in each situation. The reader is advised always to check product information (package inserts) for changes and new information regarding dose and contraindications before administering any drug. Caution is especially urged when using new or infrequently ordered drugs.

**Library of Congress Cataloging-in-Publication Data**

Carroll, Charles, 1949–
    Legal issues and ethical dilemmas in respiratory care / Charles Carroll.
      p.    cm.
    Includes bibliographical references and index.
    ISBN 0-8036-0126-3
    1. Respiratory therapy—Moral and ethical aspects.    2. Respiratory therapy—Law and legislation—United States.    I. Title.
RC735.I5C37    1996
$174'.2$—dc20                                                                           95-44083
                                                                                                                                   CIP

Authorization to photocopy items for internal or personal use, or the internal or personal use of specific clients, is granted by F. A. Davis Company for users registered with the Copyright Clearance Center (CCC) Transactional Reporting Service, provided that the fee of \$.10 per copy is paid directly to CCC, 222 Rosewood Drive, Danvers, MA 01923. For those organizations that have been granted a photocopy license by CCC, a separate system of payment has been arranged. The fee code for users of the Transactional Reporting Service is: 8036-0126/0 + \$.10.

**For Leigh, Courtney, and Neci**

# *Preface*

As health care team members, respiratory care practitioners are specialists in the evaluation, treatment, and care of patients with breathing disorders. These specialists perform their duties in physician's offices, patient homes, clinics, skilled nursing facilities, and hospitals. A 1992 Human Resource Survey conducted by the American Association for Respiratory Care (AARC), the professional organization representing respiratory care practitioners nationally, found that more than 80,000 practitioners were currently employed in the nation's hospitals. It is believed that an additional 40,000 practitioners are employed in other settings, making the total number of practitioners well over 100,000.

On a daily basis these practitioners deliver a wide array of services to patients ranging from premature infants to the elderly. Services range from treatments designed to provide temporary relief from breathing difficulties to life support for those who are unable to sustain respirations on their own. Patients suffering from chronic diseases and traumatic injuries receive therapy from respiratory care practitioners. Patients recovering from surgery and respiratory or cardiac arrest depend on respiratory care practitioners for life support services. The near drowning victim, the AIDS patient, the poststroke patient, the cystic fibrosis patient, and patients with chronic obstructive or restrictive pulmonary diseases all benefit from the many complex and specialized therapy modalities delivered by respiratory care practitioners.

In addition to therapy and treatments, respiratory care practitioners are involved in diagnostic, educational, and rehabilitation services. Diagnostic pulmonary function testing, stress testing, and arterial blood gas data are all used to make decisions concerning treatment and in some cases payment for medical services. Long- and short-term rehabilitation, educational services on pulmonary health and disease, and smoking cessation are also among the varied services performed by respiratory care practitioners.

While delivering services and providing patient care, respiratory care practitioners must be continuously aware of the legal and ethical implications of the services they deliver and their actions while delivering them. Poor or un-informed decisions can result in disastrous results for the patient, the practitioner, and the health care facility. The critical nature of health care today, the expectations of patients, the limited resources, the technological explosion, and the charged legal environment all combine to create a work setting that is highly stressful for respiratory care practitioners.

The purpose of this book is to provide respiratory care practitioners the basic information and a framework for understanding legal issues and for making ethical decisions while delivering respiratory care services. The book is not a "how-to" manual since every situation is unique and will require a solution that is also unique. However, using the ethical decision-making processes described in this book along with the applications learned from the applied activities and case studies, the respiratory care practitioner will be significantly better prepared to function as a safe professional in accordance with legal and ethical guidelines. An additional bonus will be a reduction of stress and burnout and an increase in confidence associated with making patient-care decisions.

In order to fulfill the purposes of this book, the reader is introduced to both the traditional and contemporary ethical theories and principles. The historical documents that are the foundations of many of the current ethical codes are introduced and discussed as appropriate. An entire chapter on the legal basis of respiratory care is presented as a primer on the legal status of the profession. Finally, selected topics such as confidentiality, caring for selected difficult patients, allocation of resources, advance directives, and caring for the dying patient are covered in separate chapters. Three ethical decision-making models are presented. A series of applied activities are dispersed throughout the book to assist the reader in understanding some of the concepts and in some cases in obtaining additional information applicable on a local level. Twenty case studies are included to provide examples of how some ethical situations may be resolved. An instructor's guide is available to instructors to assist them in planning class sessions and leading discussions.

Charles Carroll

# Acknowledgments

*The author would like to thank the following reviewers:*

**Thomas A. Barnes, EdD, RRT**
Associate Professor of
　Cardiopulmonary Sciences
Northeastern University
Mashfield, Massachusetts

**Anita C. Brannon, JD**
Private Practice
Tampa, Florida

**Walter C. Chop, MS, RRT**
Program Director
Respiratory Therapy
Southern Maine Technical College
South Portland, Maine

**Martha DeSilva, BS, RRT**
Director of Respiratory Care
Massasoit Community College
Carver, Massachusetts

**Raymond Scott Edge, EdD**
Associate Dean
College of Allied Health Sciences
Ferris State University
Big Rapids, Michigan

**Lyle Engstrom, BS, MA, RRT**
Program Chair
Southeast Community College
Lincoln, Nebraska

**Jackie L. Long, MEd, RRT**
Program Director
Respiratory Care Program
Newburg College
Brookline, Massachusetts

**Stanley M. Pearson, MSEd, RRT, C-CPT (NSCPT)**
Assistant Professor/Coordinator
Respiratory Therapy
Southern Illinois University
College of Technical Careers
Carbondale, Illinois

**Yvonne Jo Robbins, MEd, RRT**
Program Director
Respiratory Care Program
Westchester University/Bryn Mawr
　Hospital
Bryn Mawr, Pennsylvania

**Milton Schwartzberg, JD**
Private Practice
Boston, Massachusetts

**Robert L. Wilkins, RRT**
Associate Professor
Loma Linda University
Loma Linda, California

# Contents

How to Use This Book .................................... xv

## Part One  Foundations and Issues

*Chapter 1. An Introduction to Legal Issues and Ethical*
  *Dilemmas in Respiratory Care* ........................ 3
A Brief History of Legal Issues and Ethical Dilemmas in Health Care ..... 5
The Significance of Legal Issues and Ethical Dilemmas for Respiratory Care
  Practitioners ........................................ 9
Case Study 1 ........................................... 10
Case Study 2 ........................................... 11

*Chapter 2: Legal Regulation and Issues in*
  *Respiratory Care* .................................. 12
Introduction to the American Legal System ...................... 12
The Legal Basis for Respiratory Care Practice .................... 18
Potential Liability in Respiratory Care Practice .................. 24

*Chapter 3: Ethics and Health Care* ...................... 30
Definitions of Ethics .................................... 30
The Foundation of Ethical Thinking ........................... 31
Health, Disease, and Ethics ................................ 33
Who Is Entitled to Health Care? ............................. 36
Health Care Versus Disease Care ............................. 37
The Role of Ethics in Health Care ........................... 38

xi

*Chapter 4: The Ethical Decision-Making Process* .......... 41
The Basis of Ethical Decisions ................................ 41
Who Makes Ethical Decisions? ................................ 42
Participating in Ethical Decision Making ....................... 44

*Chapter 5: Ethical Principles* ............................. 51
Ethical Principles: The Basis of Health Care Ethics ................ 51
Differing Views of Ethical Principles: Traditional
  Versus Contemporary ..................................... 51
Traditional and Contemporary Ethical Principles and Their Meanings ..... 52
A Patient's Bill of Rights ................................... 62

*Chapter 6: Ethical Theories and Methods* ................. 68
The Deontological Theory ................................... 69
The Utilitarian Theory ...................................... 72
The Analysis Method ....................................... 74

*Chapter 7: Applied Ethical Decision Making* ............... 79
Case Study 3 .............................................. 79
Case Study 4 .............................................. 84
Case Study 5 .............................................. 86
Discussion ................................................ 87

# Part Two: *Applications and Practices*

*Chapter 8: Confidentiality* .............................. 90
The Issue ................................................. 90
Legal Considerations ....................................... 92
Ethical Considerations ..................................... 95
Case Study 6 .............................................. 95
Case Study 7 .............................................. 96

*Chapter 9: Human Experimentation and the Use
  of New Technology* ..................................... 98
The Issue ................................................. 98
Legal Considerations ....................................... 101
Ethical Considerations ..................................... 102
Case Study 8 .............................................. 103

*Chapter 10: Dealing With Difficult Patients* ............... 105
The Issue ................................................. 105
Legal Considerations ....................................... 109

Ethical Considerations ..................................... 110
Therapeutic Communication ................................ 110
Case Study 9 ................................................ 111

## Chapter 11: Caring for Patients With Chronic Illness or Communicable Diseases ........................... 113
The Issue .................................................... 113
Legal Considerations ....................................... 115
Ethical Considerations ..................................... 115
Guidelines for Delivery of Care ............................ 116
Case Study 10 ............................................... 117
Case Study 11 ............................................... 118

## Chapter 12: Caring for the Terminally Ill and Dying Patient ................................... 121
The Issue .................................................... 121
Legal Considerations ....................................... 126
Ethical Considerations ..................................... 128
Case Study 12 ............................................... 130

## Chapter 13: Advance Directives ........................ 133
The Issue .................................................... 133
Legal Considerations ....................................... 136
Ethical Considerations ..................................... 139
Case Study 13 ............................................... 140

## Chapter 14: Allocation of Resources ................... 142
The Issue .................................................... 142
Legal Considerations ....................................... 145
Ethical Considerations ..................................... 146
Case Study 14 ............................................... 147

## Chapter 15: A Closing Perspective ..................... 150
The Importance of Studying Legal Issues and Ethical Dilemmas ........ 150
The Importance of Studying Critical Thinking and Systematic
  Decision Making ......................................... 151
Case Study 15 ............................................... 154
Case Study 16 ............................................... 155
Case Study 17 ............................................... 155

## Index ..................................................... 159

# *How to Use This Book*

The design of this book allows for its use as a classroom textbook, as a supplement to a clinical course, or as a guide for independent study. As a classroom textbook, the 15 chapters fit well in a semester or quarter term with 12 to 15 weeks. Students may be assigned a chapter per week, or in the case of shorter terms, two or more of the shorter chapters may be assigned for 1 week. Class time should be spent reviewing the key concepts in each chapter, reviewing the applied activities, and discussing the case studies. Students should be challenged to participate in discussions by including current event information from journals and newspapers that relate to the topics under discussion.

This book is an excellent supplement to a clinical course in those cases where an instructor cannot expand the already limited lecture time. Assignments to the students would be similar to those in the classroom settings. Discussions would be held as part of the preclinical and postclinical conference activities. A major advantage to this method is that the material will be discussed while in the patient care setting. This should bring a sense of realism that may not be present in the classroom setting.

Finally, this book will provide insightful reading and information to any practitioner who decides to read it on his or her own as part of personal professional development. As respiratory care practitioners continue to strive to be recognized as the full professionals that they are, knowledge and awareness of legal and ethical issues are essential elements that must be grasped.

# PART ONE

# Foundations and Issues

# CHAPTER 1

# *An Introduction to Legal Issues and Ethical Dilemmas in Respiratory Care*

**A Brief History of Legal Issues and Ethical Dilemmas in Health Care**
From No Risk to Risk Management
From the Hippocratic Oath to Professional Codes of Ethics
**The Significance of Legal Issues and Ethical Dilemmas for Respiratory Care Practitioners**
Common Legal Issues in Respiratory Care
Common Ethical Dilemmas in Respiratory Care
**Case Studies**
Case Study 1: Legal Issues
Case Study 2: Ethical Dilemmas

Avoiding legal and ethical pitfalls is not usually the foremost concern of respiratory care practitioners. Since most practitioners are well trained, conscientious, and professional, the care of patients is the primary concern. Most practitioners would never take any action that would knowingly result in any mental or physical harm or discomfort to a patient. Yet, in the routine delivery of care, respiratory care practitioners encounter many potential legal and ethical snarls. Consider the following scenarios.

*Case Study #1: Legal Scenario*

Jon Apple is a respiratory care practitioner in the state of Florida. He works alone in a small community hospital on the 11-to-7 shift. He attends school during the day working toward a degree in health care management. His long-term goal is to become a respiratory therapy department head. As a result of a heavy class load and a busy personal life, Jon is not getting adequate sleep. And so, Monday night at work after a long day of classes and a busy weekend, Jon locks the door to the department, sets the alarm on his watch for 15 minutes, props his feet on the desk, and closes his eyes. Before closing his eyes, Jon notes the time. It is 1:30 AM. Minutes earlier, he had checked every respiratory patient in the hospital and taken care of their needs. Both the intensive care unit and the emergency room are now quiet, and the staff is bored and browsing through magazines. Surely, Jon wouldn't be needed for another hour. However, he wanted only 15 minutes to "rest" his eyes—he did not plan to go to sleep, and he *knew* he would hear the beeper or pager if needed.

Jon woke to the sound of banging on the department door. Rubbing the sleep from his eyes, he quickly unlocked the door. The nursing supervisor was looking for him since he had not answered his beeper or responded to the code that had been called 45 minutes earlier. Jon felt a sense of doom as he faced the nursing supervisor in the doorway.

---

This incident will create a major legal issue for Jon, who is a licensed respiratory care practitioner. His irresponsible actions will be reported to the supervisor and possibly to the hospital administrator. Depending on the type of disciplinary action taken against him, it is possible that the state licensing regulatory board may become involved.

The hospital also has a major risk management concern in this situation. In the code that Jon missed, it was the respiratory care practitioner's responsibility to manage the airway. Obviously, Jon was not present to carry out his duties. If the patient suffered any adverse effects at all, regardless of whether they were a direct result of Jon's absence or not, the patient's family now has a legal cause of action against the hospital. If a lawsuit is filed, Jon's failure to carry out his assigned duties would place both himself and the hospital at a legal disadvantage. Although the filing of a lawsuit does not constitute proof of legal wrongdoing, it is important not to be at a legal disadvantage if such action is taken. As illustrated in this scenario, it is extremely important for respiratory care practitioners to be aware of the potential legal implications and consequences of their actions.

*Case Study #2: Ethical Scenario*

Jan and Angel are employed by a large home care company. Their duties include seeing a large number of patients on a scheduled basis. They work independently; however, they often meet for lunch and sometimes after work. Jan notices that during their planned meetings, Angel often spends time completing her patients' logs. Company policy, in an attempt to maintain quality control, requires that the logs be completed before leaving the patient's house. Company experience has shown that when logs are completed later, the number of inaccuracies increases dramatically.

Jan's concern, however, goes beyond Angel's violation of company policy. She suspects that Angel is actually fabricating some of the patients' logs. Her suspicion is based on several factors. Angel regularly tells Jan about going shopping or about stopping at home to watch her favorite television show. Occasionally, Jan detects an odor of what she believes to be alcohol on Angel's breath when they meet. Angel always dismisses Jan's questions about her patients with a flippant remark.

One day Jan observes Angel's car parked in the parking lot of a popular mall for over 2 hours. When they meet later for lunch, Angel completes patients' logs for the same time frame. Jan has a dilemma. Although she does not have absolute proof that Angel is falsifying records, she is convinced that her suspicions are justified. She feels that the only way to obtain absolute proof is to inform the supervisor of her suspicions and have the supervisor investigate.

---

The ethical dilemma faced by Jan is similar to those faced by respiratory care practitioners on a regular basis. Dilemmas exist whenever there are two somewhat equally desirable or undesirable choices. In this scenario, Jan is faced with two undesirable choices. She can either ignore the situation, possibly resulting in patients not receiving the care they deserve, or she can report her suspicions to her supervisor, starting a chain of events that could result in serious trouble for her friend Angel. Ultimately, Jan will decide which is the lesser evil. She will arrive at this decision by appraising the value she assigns to certain ethical principles. Jan may be unaware of the systematic decision-making process available to her and as a result experience a significant amount of unnecessary distress in the process. Afterward she may wonder if her choice was correct.

Later in this book, we present several systematic decision-making processes that may be used when dealing with ethical dilemmas. First, however, a historical overview of legal issues and ethical dilemmas in health care may be helpful.

## A BRIEF HISTORY OF LEGAL ISSUES AND ETHICAL DILEMMAS IN HEALTH CARE

In colonial America, health care providers were faced with few legal issues and probably even fewer known ethical dilemmas. The education and practice of early American health care providers, primarily physicians, reflected the individualistic mood of the times. Medical training was conducted through apprenticeships by which an aspiring physician simply teamed with an experienced doctor and learned the trade of medicine under the guidance of the mentor.

In 1752, Pennsylvania Hospital, the first major American hospital, opened in Philadelphia. Shortly after that, the hospital developed a formalized apprenticeship program and by 1756 had founded a medical school. King's College, which later became Columbia University, opened the second medical school in 1768. In 1783, Harvard University established a medical school. Dartmouth College followed the lead of the other three schools and began to offer medical training in 1797. Thus, by 1800, formal training in medicine was becoming a reality. However, effective licensure procedures were still a future event. In 1821, Georgia became the first state to require graduation from a medical school as a condition of licensure. This act was taken in the midst of ongoing upheaval over the licensing of physicians in general. Apprentice-trained physicians generally opposed licensure. Despite this opposition, the movement toward formal education and effective licensing procedures continued. Although many major changes have occurred since then, by 1900 the framework for our current medical education and licensing system was in effect.[1]

Historically, formal professional training for respiratory care practitioners has closely paralleled that of physicians. Starting with on-the-job, or informal apprenticeship training, the profession has evolved from primarily hospital-based schools to primarily college- and university-based schools. Credentialing has evolved from none at all to national certification and registration to the current requirement of licensure in most states.

## From No Risk to Risk Management

Early health care practitioners had little concern over being sued for malpractice. Practitioners were generally held in high esteem, and mistakes were dismissed as unfortunate events. It was unthinkable to question the practitioner's judgment. Over the years, however, patients' attitudes changed. By the mid-1980s, one out of every ten physicians had some type of malpractice claim filed against him or her.[2] The risk is continuing to increase, and larger and larger jury awards of damages make the cost of liability insurance and defensive medicine one of the most expensive components of providing health care.

As a result of the "deep pocket" theory of suing the entity most capable of paying, it is the physicians, hospitals, and drug companies that are most commonly sued. However, as respiratory care practitioners and other allied health care personnel become more involved in offering various specialized health care services, personal liability for these practitioners is also increasing. Luckily for hospital-employed practitioners, some liability insurance is provided by the employer. For practitioners who work as independent contractors or on an as-needed basis, liability insurance may be simply a necessary business expense.

In addition to maintaining liability insurance for their financial protection, larger hospitals and other health care institutions now have fully staffed risk management departments. The risk manager's job is twofold. The first task is to eliminate or reduce any possible risk the hospital might encounter. This is done by reviewing policies, procedures, and actions of personnel and eliminating those which have a high probability of putting the hospital at risk for a lawsuit. The second task is to minimize the amount of money that the institution must pay to defend itself if a lawsuit is filed. Training and certification are available in some states for certified risk managers. Thus, although it once fared little or no risk, the health care industry now does not question the existence of risk but looks to ways risk can best be managed. Respiratory care practitioners must be cognitive of this evolution and prepared to function effectively and safely in the current dynamic legal climate.

## From the Hippocratic Oath to Professional Codes of Ethics

The modern practice of healing has always carried with it the aura of being a noble calling. Practitioners were seen as unselfish individuals who placed the well-being of their patients above their personal well-being. Ethical behavior was loosely based on the Hippocratic oath (Box 1-1). This ancient document has had a profound impact on the practice of healing. It is the basis for modern-day codes of ethics adopted by many of the healing professions.

### Box 1–1. THE HIPPOCRATIC OATH*

"I swear by Apollo Physician, by Asclepius, by Health, by Panacea, and by all the gods and goddesses, making them my witnesses, that I will carry out, according to my ability and judgment, this oath and this indenture. To hold my teacher in this art equal to my own parents; to make him partner in my livelihood; when he is in need of money to share mine with him; to consider his family as my own brothers, and to teach them this art, if they want to learn it, without fee or indenture.

"To impart precept, oral instruction, and all other instruction to my own sons, the sons of my teacher, and to indentured pupils who have taken the physicians's oath, but to nobody else. I will use treatment to help the sick according to my ability and judgment, but never with a view to injury and wrongdoing. Neither will I administer a poison to anybody when asked to do so, nor will I suggest such a course. Similarly, I will not give to a woman a pessary to cause abortion. But I will keep pure and holy both my life and my art.

"I will not use the knife, no even, verily, on sufferers from stone, but I will give place to such as are craftsmen therein. Into whatsoever houses I enter, I will enter to help the sick, and I will abstain from all intentional wrongdoing and harm, especially from abusing the bodies of man or woman, bond or free.

"And whatsoever I shall see or hear in the course of my profession, as well as outside my profession in my intercourse with men, it be what should not be published abroad, I will never divulge, holding such things to be holy secrets.

"Now, if I carry out this oath, break it not, may I gain forever reputation among all men for my life and for my art; but if I transgress it and forswear myself, may the opposite befall me."

*From Hippocrates. The Oath. In Hippocrates, vol 1 (translated by W.H.S. Jones, The Loeb Classic Library). Harvard University Press, Cambridge, MA, 1923, pp 299–301.

Hippocrates, a Greek physician who lived from around 460 BC to 349 BC, is widely acclaimed to be responsible for the Hippocratic oath, but there is some debate as to how much of the oath he actually wrote. The oath was adopted by early physicians and for a while was recited by new physicians during their graduation ceremony from medical school. The practice has since diminished significantly. For a time, the oath embodied the great and noble aspirations embodied by the practicing physician, focusing on the physician's duty to the patient and to other members of the medical profession. It was also restrictive, having within it clear prohibitions against abortion and euthanasia. At least two of the charges given in the oath are still very much a part of the ethical and legal codes observed by health care professions today: the need to maintain confidentiality and the dictum not to use the care giver–patient relationship to influence a patient to engage in sexual activities.[3]

Although the Hippocratic oath is no longer the sole defining document for the ethical conduct of health care practitioners, many components of the oath form the basis for the ethical codes adopted by many health professions. Common components found in the Hippocratic oath as well as the ethical codes adopted by other health care professions include emphasis on ability, not causing harm to patients, confidentiality, and proper sexual conduct. The American Association for Respiratory Care (AARC) has adopted a code of ethics for respiratory care practitioners (Box 1–2). Some states have adopted this code as part of their respiratory care acts. The AARC has also developed a set of protocols and clinical guidelines to assist the practitioner in delivering quality care. Attention to these guidelines will assist the practitioner in complying with the code of ethics.

---

**Box 1–2. THE AMERICAN ASSOCIATION FOR RESPIRATORY CARE'S STATEMENT OF ETHICS AND PROFESSIONAL CONDUCT***

*In the conduct of their professional activities the Respiratory Care Practitioner shall be bound by the following ethical and professional principles. Respiratory Care Practitioners shall:*

- Demonstrate behavior that reflects integrity, supports objectivity, and fosters trust in the profession and its professionals.
- Actively maintain and continually improve their professional competence, and represent it accurately.
- Perform only those procedures or functions in which they are individually competent and which are within the scope of accepted and responsible practice.
- Respect and protect the legal and personal rights of patients they treat, including the right to informed consent and refusal of treatment.
- Divulge no confidential information regarding any patient or family unless disclosure is required for responsible performance of duty, or required by law.
- Provide care without discrimination on any basis, with respect for the rights and dignity of all individuals.
- Promote disease prevention and wellness.
- Refuse to participate in illegal or unethical acts, and shall refuse to conceal illegal, unethical or incompetent acts of others.
- Follow sound scientific procedures and ethical principles in research.
- Comply with state or federal laws which govern and relate to their practice.
- Avoid any form of conduct that creates a conflict of interest, and shall follow the principles of ethical business behavior.
- Promote the positive evolution of the profession, and health care in general, through improvement of the access, efficacy, and cost of patient care.
- Refrain from indiscriminate and unnecessary use of resources, both economic and natural, in their practice.

*From the American Association for Respiratory Care: Statement of Ethics and Professional Conduct. AARC Times, February 1995, p 72, with permission.

# THE SIGNIFICANCE OF LEGAL ISSUES AND ETHICAL DILEMMAS FOR RESPIRATORY CARE PRACTITIONERS

Providing care for sick persons is a rewarding experience, but the responsibility of providing such care is grave. The patient's ability to breathe, the most critical life function, is often dependent on the knowledge and skill of the respiratory care practitioner. Failure to comply with the legal and ethical responsibilities associated with providing such care can result in serious consequences for both the patient and the practitioner.

## Common Legal Issues in Respiratory Care

Health care is one of the most highly regulated industries in our country. As health care providers, respiratory care practitioners must deliver their services within the boundaries of the various laws and regulations that govern the delivery of health care. Although respiratory care practitioners have not been named in lawsuits in significant numbers, they are not exempt from the need to practice within legal boundaries. Furthermore, there is no assurance that the number of respiratory care practitioners named in lawsuits will remain as low in the future as it has in the past.

The legal status of respiratory care practitioners has changed rapidly over the past decade. During the early 1980s a continuous effort to establish licensing for respiratory care practitioners began to show positive results. By early 1994, 38 states had achieved some form of legal credentialing.[4] Committees in the remaining states are working to establish similar licensing procedures. (The details of legal credentialing for respiratory care practitioners are discussed in detail in Chapter 2.)

Legal credentialing has done much to enhance the professional status of respiratory care. A further discussion of the meaning of professionalism is included in Chapter 2. Benefits, however, seldom come without responsibility. Thus, along with the many benefits of legal credentialing, practitioners also face increased legal responsibilities. Many of these legal responsibilities actually existed prior to licensing laws but are now more clearly defined. Common legal issues in respiratory care include:

1. Practicing without an appropriate license or certification
2. Falsifying or maintaining incomplete patient records
3. Performing therapy without an order
4. Conducting oneself in an unprofessional manner
5. Working while under the influence of alcohol, drugs, or narcotics
6. Practicing under the influence of a mental or physical condition that impairs the ability to deliver services with reasonable skill and safety
7. Failure to deliver therapy with a reasonable level of skill
8. Attempting to perform duties that the practitioner is not competent to perform
9. Assigning another practitioner duties to perform that the assignee is not competent to perform
10. Failure to complete required continuing education requirements
11. Therapist-driven rather than detailed physician's orders

## Common Ethical Dilemmas in Respiratory Care

Respiratory care practitioners face the same basic ethical dilemmas faced by other health care practitioners. The range of ethical dilemmas for all health care practitioners is growing rapidly every day. It should be noted that a practitioner does not have to be in a position to make a decision about an ethical dilemma in order to be affected by it. For example, although a practitioner may not have the authority to decide who will benefit from advanced technological care, if that practitioner works where such dilemmas occur, then he or she is integrally involved in an ethical dilemma. Thus, respiratory care practitioners are faced with all the ethical dilemmas that challenge health care today. Common ethical dilemmas faced by respiratory care practitioners and other health care workers include:

1. The need to protect the confidentiality of patients' records
2. The rationing of resources for patient care
3. Inadequate staffing for safe patient care
4. Inability of patients to pay for needed services
5. The presence of do not resuscitate orders
6. Incompetence on the part of fellow practitioners
7. Impaired performance by fellow practitioners
8. The challenge of caring for the dying patient
9. Caring for patients with infectious diseases such as AIDS
10. The proper use of experimental procedures

## CASE STUDIES

Case studies will be used in this text to help the reader understand how to apply the content presented in most chapters. In this chapter, the case studies used will be a continuation of the scenarios presented at the beginning of the chapter.

Case studies should be approached systematically; for some there will be no absolute correct answer or best solution. For each case study presented, answer the following questions and prepare to discuss your answers with your instructor and classmates. Your instructor may have resources that will suggest an acceptable answer or solution.

1. What problem is presented in the case study?
2. Is the problem a legal issue, an ethical dilemma, or both?
3. What legal or ethical principles apply to this problem?
4. What is the most desirable solution to this problem?

### Case Study 1: Legal Issues

> Reread the legal scenario presented at the beginning of this chapter and answer the "case study" questions. Although the case study is already identified as a legal issue, be sure to answer the second question. You also may be able to find an ethical dilemma.

## Case Study 2: Ethical Dilemmas

Reread the ethical scenario presented at the beginning of this chapter and answer the "case study" questions. Although the case study is identified as an ethical issue, be sure to answer the second question. You also may be able to find a legal issue.

## STUDY QUESTIONS

1. *What is the difference between legal issues and ethical dilemmas?*

2. *Select two of the common legal issues listed in the chapter and discuss their significance.*

3. *Select two of the common ethical issues listed in the chapter and discuss their significance.*

4. *What is the purpose of liability insurance for health care practitioners?*

5. *Name three components of the Hippocratic oath that have disappeared from most ethical codes in use today.*

## REFERENCES

1. Raffel, NK, and Raffel, MW: The U.S. Health Care System, Origins and Functions, ed 3. Delmar, Albany, NY, 1989, p 26.
2. Ibid.
3. Hippocrates. The Oath. In Hippocrates: vol I (translated by W.H.S. Jones, The Loeb Classic Library). Harvard University Press, Cambridge, MA, 1923, pp 299–301 (quote p 301).
4. Eicher, J: State credentiating update. AARC Times, March 1994.
5. American Association for Respiratory Care: Statement of Ethics and Professional Conduct, rev ed, December 1994. AARC Times, February 1995, p 72.

CHAPTER 2

# Legal Regulation and Issues in Respiratory Care

**Introduction to the American Legal System**
Sources and Types of Law
Courts and the Trial Process
**The Legal Basis for Respiratory Care Practice**
National Registration and Certification
State Respiratory Care Practice Acts
**Potential Liability in Respiratory Care Practice**
Professional Liability
Malpractice Prevention
Malpractice Protection

## INTRODUCTION TO THE AMERICAN LEGAL SYSTEM

The American legal system is extremely complex.[1] This chapter offers an overview of our legal system for respiratory care practitioners seeking to understand some of these complexities. The chapter is not intended to serve as a definitive legal manual. All the nuances of the American legal system cannot and should not be presented in a textbook focusing on the legal and ethical concerns of respiratory care. Respiratory care practitioners in need of specific legal advice should seek the services of a competent attorney.

The American legal system has its roots in early English common law. Important elements of our legal system that derive from English common law include the jury, the grand jury, professional judges, reliance on legal precedent, and appellate review of lower courts. One significant aspect of English common law that has recently seen renewed emphasis in American law is restitution. When fines were imposed for violation of English common law, the fine was paid directly to the victim rather than to a government agency. Although restitution has figured in some cases since colonial days, American criminal law has recently begun to use this concept more frequently.[2]

The largest body of laws governing our everyday life consists of statutes that are enacted on the federal level by Congress or on the state level by state legislatures. The origins of this body of laws derive from the collective moral conscience of our society. Our society's concepts of right and wrong are greatly influenced by Judeo-Christian tradition. Despite a vast sea of statutes enacted by federal and state legislative bodies, there will always be gaps that are not addressed, and in those cases most of the states look to English common law for guidance. In at least one state, Louisiana, the Napoleonic civil code rather than English common law is used to fill statutory gaps.

Generally, statutory law may be divided into two broad categories: civil law and criminal law. Civil law addresses dealings among citizens, governmental entities, and corporations. Civil lawsuits typically involve disputes over contracts or compensation for injuries and damages by one party to another. Criminal law addresses offenses against the state, which initiates the legal action. Criminal law statutes address specific rights and wrongs and are accompanied by specified punishment, ranging from incarceration or even capital punishment in the most severe cases to fines in the least severe cases.

Although these legislatively enacted statutes provide the major guidelines for behavior that is permitted under our Constitution, there are modes of behavior that cannot or should not be regulated by law, particularly in a free society. This was recognized by Alexis DeTocqueville when he stated: "There is no country in the world in which everything can be provided for by the laws, or in which political institutions can provide a substitute for common sense and public morality."[3]

In recent years, specific groups of persons, disciplines, and professional associations have deemed it necessary to formulate ethical guidelines. Principles that provide guidelines for behavior in the area of ethical conduct are on a plane well below conduct regulated by law. In some cases, professional practice acts have incorporated the professional association's code of ethics as part of the statute. In those cases, ethical misconduct could conceivably be equivalent to a criminal violation of law.

Another view of the relationship between ethics and law is illustrated by a continuum devised by the author showing how personal values may become either a law or a principle of ethical behavior (Table 2–1).

## Sources and Types of Laws

As average citizens conduct their routine affairs, they may be affected by laws from many different sources. Various governmental entities have the authority to develop and to enforce laws within certain established boundaries. The Constitution of the United States sets forth the framework of government in this country, and it also imposes certain limitations on its citizens. Although the Constitution gives broad police powers to the states, it does not directly mention either medicine or health.[4]

**Table 2–1.** THE ETHICS–LAW CONTINUUM

- *Law*—When elected representatives of a society are called upon to crystallize or legislate what constitutes legal behavior, we see a manifestation of the society's values in the resulting legislation. There may, however, be disagreement among members of society as to the validity of a given law.
- *Ethics*—When microcosms of the same society deem it necessary to establish a moral code of behavior, or ethics, for members of their group, discipline, profession, etc., those ethics are drawn from the same moral values that pervade the microcosm. Ethical codes fill a gap that is not addressed by legal statutes, as most often it is the groups that impose compliance with their particular code of ethics as a condition of membership. The codes generally do not attempt to address behavior already addressed by legal statutes, though there is invariably some overlap. Likewise, legal statutes generally do not attempt to address areas of behavior that are more appropriately addressed by ethical codes or have no restraints at all. The Hippocratic oath taken by physicians is an example of an ethical code which has been in use for over 2000 years.
- *Societal Values*—A society's "sense" of right and wrong is a product of its culture, which in turn is formulated over time by the customs and practices of those who make up the society. The value system of any given society is difficult to quantify when looking in from the outside, and there is likely to be variation in values from individual to individual.

The Constitution is a dynamic document. Twenty-six amendments have been added to it over the years. In fact, one of the most commonly quoted parts of the Constitution is the First Amendment, which among other things, guarantees freedom of speech. This amendment is open to interpretation, which is subject to change, as views of society change with the passage of time. While the Constitution imposes limitations upon the government and the laws it may enact, the Congress and the state legislatures (the legislative branch of government) have the greatest impact on our daily lives by means of numerous statutes that have been enacted over the years. These numerous laws determine such things as how much tax we pay and how the cost of health care will be reimbursed.

In addition to the Constitution of the United States, each of the 50 states also has a state constitution and its own governmental framework, which for the most part mimics the federal system. Each state also has a legislative, a judicial, and an executive branch of government. Some counties and cities have charters, or constitutions that define their governmental framework and their own legislative bodies that adopt ordinances applicable to the particular local government, but this varies throughout the country.

Regulatory agencies have also acquired quasi-legislative authority. Many areas of the law have resulted from an enactment by a legislature which expresses the intent to oversee a particular aspect of governmental authority, such as taxation. On the federal level, Congress has enacted statutes regarding taxation and has expressed its intent regarding taxation. In doing so, Congress has authorized the Internal Revenue Service to promulgate regulations which carry out the intent of the statutes enacted by the Congress. In these cases, we see the executive branch exercising both its constitutional authority to enforce laws as well as a quasi-legislative authority to promulgate regulations consistent with the enabling act passed by Congress. Utilization of executive agencies in this fashion carries down to the state and local governmental levels as well. This is just one example of the workings of regulatory agencies and their impact on the law. The exceptions and variations are too numerous to mention here.

For the most part, laws with the greatest impact on respiratory care practitioners are either federal or state. In the daily delivery of respiratory care services, federal law has its greatest impact on reimbursement, drugs, and medical devices. Other federal agencies and entities such as the Centers for Disease Control, the Food and Drug Administration, National Institutes of Health, and the Surgeon General's office may impact the delivery of respiratory care services. These are all agencies of the executive branch of government. State law impacts reimbursement as well as the administrative operation of health care facilities and the credentialing of health care professionals.

Although there are several ways of classifying law, we discuss only two: law classified according to its source (federal, state, or local) and law classified according to its application (civil or criminal). As discussed earlier, civil law consists of those laws which govern affairs between private individuals, governmental agencies, or entities. In criminal law, the offense is against the public, and the state initiates and carries out the legal action.

Because state law has more of a specific day-to-day impact on respiratory care practitioners, this discussion focuses on laws enacted at that level. Each state has a legislative body that enacts statutory law. The statutes are often broad in scope and do not contain all the details necessary for application of that law, and, as in the example of federal regulatory law previously given, states have established agencies under the executive branch to enforce the law and to authorize each agency to promulgate regulations which enforce the intent of the legislative body in more detail.

The Respiratory Care Practice Act is an example of a uniform act that many states have adopted in an effort to regulate the practice of respiratory care. An agency or a board or council of respiratory care may be designated to administer the act. The responsibility of this body would be to enforce the statutes, that is, the practice act, enacted by the legislature. In addition, this body would be responsible for enforcing its own regulations which are developed within the parameters of intent embodied in the statue enacted by the legislature.

Conduct that the legislature has deemed criminal must be clearly defined so as to comply with the constitutional requirement precluding vagueness. While the accompanying regulatory scheme may impose fines for certain misconduct expressed in the legislation, regulatory agency authority does not extend to defining criminal acts. While agencies do have quasi-legislative authority, defining criminal acts within that authority would clearly exceed the separation-of-powers concept of the Constitution, which limits the executive branch to enforcement of laws.

Civil law deals primarily with the legal relationship between entities. The entities may be individuals, e.g., two citizens, a health care worker and a patient, small businesses, and large corporations or organizations. Generally, in a civil case, one entity (a plaintiff) will bring legal action against another entity (the defendant) to obtain redress (relief) for a perceived wrong. The forum with jurisdiction to hear the matter serves as an impartial fact finder, applies applicable law to those facts, and in so doing decides the case. Generally, wrongs are addressed in civil cases by one of two methods. Normally, monetary damages will be sought by the plaintiff, and in rare cases where monetary damages would be insufficient, some type of equitable relief may be sought. Equitable relief is that which is just and conforms to the principles of justice and right (see Box 2–1). In even fewer cases, both monetary and equitable relief may be appropriate. Other forms of relief are available, but a discussion of them is beyond the scope of this chapter.

In many courts, corporations are required to be represented by an attorney, but it is not always necessary in the case of individuals. Given the highly complex nature of legal proceedings in this day and time, the oft-quoted maxim: "Only a fool represents himself as a client" is understandable.

When a patient brings legal action against a health care facility or health care worker, it is generally for the reason that he or she claims to have suffered some injury as a result of negligence on the part of the defendants. The patient (plaintiff) carries the burden of showing that something happened out of the ordinary that was a breach of duty of care owed by the defendant and the burden of also proving injury of loss that is compensable by money damages. Although there may be variations from jurisdiction to jurisdiction, the burden of proof is usually by the "greater weight of the evidence." For example, when scales are equally balanced on both sides and then a feather is placed on one side, the greater weight of the evidence would be on the side of the feather. It is enough to tip the scales ever so slightly to one side or the other. The tribunal may be a single judge or a jury. Generally speaking, plaintiffs have a right of trial by jury.

---

### Box 2–1. EXAMPLE OF EQUITABLE RELIEF

A respiratory care practitioner accepts employment with Company X. The company places the practitioner in a 500-bed hospital to deliver respiratory care services pursuant to a contract between the hospital and Company X. At the time of accepting employment with Company X, the practitioner signs a contract that contains a not-to-compete covenant. In the event that the company loses its contract with the hospital, this covenant prohibits the practitioner from being employed by the hospital for a 2-year period. Company X then loses its contract, and the practitioner accepts employment with the hospital. Company X brings suit on its contract alleging that the practitioner is violating the terms of the contract. The court grants injunctive relief to Company X by prohibiting the practitioner from continuing employment at that hospital for a period of 2 years.

Legislatures establish certain laws designed to ensure the safety of and promote the welfare of the public. When these laws are broken, the consequences may range from a fine to incarceration to even death (in the event of a capital offense). The alleged law breaker, often called the defendant, is charged with the offense by the city, county, state, or federal government, which is charged with the responsibility for enforcing the law it claims has been violated. Sometimes the governmental entity is referred to as "the people." Legal representation is provided to the governmental entity by a district or state attorney or solicitor general, depending on the structure of the governmental entity involved. The "people's attorney," generally called the prosecuting attorney, is often an elected official. Although the governmental entity prosecutes the case, the actual victim is usually an individual citizen, for example, in the crimes of theft, rape, or murder. It should always be remembered that anyone charged with a criminal offense is presumed to be innocent until his or her guilt is established beyond a reasonable doubt. This is a much higher burden of proof than required in civil cases.

Violations of criminal law are classified as a misdemeanor or a felony, and within these two classifications are subdivisions, such as first-degree felony. Misdemeanors may involve nonviolent or less serious violent offenses, and if money is involved, the amount is limited. Examples of misdemeanors include disorderly conduct, petit theft, and shoplifting. Felonies, on the other hand, are serious offenses such as murder, arson, bank robbery, robberies with a gun, and drug trafficking. Generally, to establish the commission of a criminal act, one must show that it was an intentional and deliberate act on the part of the perpetrator, that is, that the perpetrator had criminal intent. There are some exceptions, for example, driving under the influence of alcohol.

One would presume that a respiratory care practitioner would not often face criminal justice issues; however, acts such as falsifying records or even failing to disclose information on an application for licensure to practice respiratory care or other professions may constitute fraud or perjury, both of which could result in criminal charges.

Criminal penalties span a wide range of possibilities. One convicted of a crime may be required to pay a fine, perform community service, pay restitution to the victim, spend time on probation, or serve time in jail—or some combination of these. In some states, the death penalty may be invoked for a particularly heinous crime like murder.

## Courts and the Trial Process

Once a legal action is started, whether civil or criminal, the judicial branch of government—the court system—becomes involved. The American judicial system is complex. One way of classifying the various courts is to look at the authority that limits the particular court's jurisdiction. Using this method, courts can be classified as local, state, or federal. As with laws, the courts also vary considerably among the states. The following descriptions are generalized. The lowest level of state courts may have names like municipal court, traffic court, juvenile court, or small claims court. The authority of these courts is limited to a specific area and to crimes or violations of a specific nature. These courts may also be referred to as city or county courts but are often actually lower-level state courts.

The names of the different levels of state courts vary from state to state. However, all states generally have one or two trial court levels and one or more appellate courts that may review the decisions of the lower courts. The trial courts have broad jurisdiction over state and civil actions. The appellate court reviews decisions of the trial court or the lower appellate court. Appellate review is undertaken only if an appeal is filed or initiated by a legal entity or authority. Who can file an appeal and under what circumstances an appeal may be filed are both subjects of other complex rules.

Each state has a supreme court that serves two functions. First, it is the final court of appeal for review of decisions made in the lower state courts. Second, it decides those cases which require an interpretation of the state constitution of state law. It may also determine some cases involving U.S. constitutional issues; however, it is not the court of last resort in those cases. Civil trials vary considerably in that a plaintiff usually contends that a defendant has committed a breach of a duty or a breach of contract which caused some harm to the plaintiff and the plaintiff is seeking to recover damages for that perceived wrong. In nearly all civil cases the type of redress sought is financial. Equitable relief, such as discussed previously, may also be sought in a civil case.

On the other hand, in a criminal trial, a governmental entity (city, county, state, or federal) is the plaintiff who contends that the defendant has violated some law that it must enforce. Although at times financial restitution to the victim is sought, the primary purposes of the criminal system is to punish those convicted of crimes. The punishment is viewed as a deterrent to future criminal behavior.

## THE LEGAL BASIS FOR RESPIRATORY CARE PRACTICE

Respiratory care has traditionally been practiced as an extension of the authority given physicians by the local state medical practice act. This is a traditional mechanism used by physicians to extend the delivery of medical services in areas other than respiratory care. Many new medical professions were initially developed using this mechanism. Some medical professions still use this mechanism to establish authority to deliver services to patients. Under this mechanism, the only legal concerns for the respiratory care practitioner were whether he or she had an appropriate order from a duly licensed physician and the appropriate competency to carry out the order. The first legal concern was generally taken care of by the hospital's credentialing system for medical staff members. The second concern, the appropriateness of the order, was taken care of by hospital standards, policy and procedure, and physician peer review. However, a knowledge base and the judgment of the respiratory care practitioner played a role in this second concern. Theoretically, the second concern might also be taken care of by the hiring and supervisory process of the hospital.

The legal doctrine that covers the relationship between physicians and respiratory care practitioners is called *respondeat superior*. This Latin phrase means "let the master answer." This doctrine holds that the person with the superior knowledge, the physician (the master), is responsible for the actions of the respiratory care practitioner (the servant). As in all employer-employee relationships, this doctrine applies directly if the respiratory care practitioner is an employee of the physician. The doctrine also applies under a variation called the "borrowed servant."

The borrowed servant variation developed because the respiratory care practitioner is employed by the hospital for the sole purpose of being "loaned" to the physician to carry out the orders written by the physician. While this loan arrangement does not free the hospital from all liability for the respiratory care practitioner's action, it does place the physician in a direct line of liability. Since the respiratory care practitioner can provide patient care only on the order of the physician, then the physician assumes the power and right to control the activities of the respiratory care practitioner. As a result, a quasi employer-employee relationship is developed.

Although respiratory care practitioners are legally responsible for their acts of negligence, both the hospital and the physician may also be held liable under the doctrine of *respondeat superior*. Liability clearly exists so long as the respiratory care practitioner's actions are within the scope of instructions given and the job description. Once the respiratory care practitioner steps beyond this scope, the hospital's and the physician's liability becomes less clearly defined. The deciding factor for liability may rest on the issue of whether the hospital or physician could reasonably have foreseen or predicted the adverse action by the respiratory care practitioner.

A topic closely related to the legal status of respiratory care practitioners is the issue of the professional status of these practitioners. From a general view, our society may think of a professional as anyone who performs a job with a positive attitude and a high level of competence. The complexity of the job may or may not be considered. There is, however, a legal definition of the professional employee which was developed by Public Law 93 360 in 1974. The intent was to define professionalism for the purposes of collective bargaining. The definition is contained in Box 2–2.

## National Registration and Certification

Respiratory care practitioners in all 50 states are eligible for registration and certification from the National Board for Respiratory Care (NBRC) if they meet certain educational requirements. Graduates of 2- or 4-year schools are eligible for the Registered Respiratory Therapist (RRT) credential. Graduates of 1-year programs are eligible for the Certified Respiratory Therapy Technician (CRTT) credential.

Registration and certification serve as a measure of competency of respiratory care practitioners, although it does not carry the weight of licensure. Hospitals and other employers can be assured that a practitioner who holds one of these credentials has received a certain level of training and at some point passed a standardized examination. The actual competency of the practitioner can usually be ascertained by interviewing the practitioner or evaluating his or her clinical performance.

> **Box 2–2. PROFESSIONALISM AS DEFINED BY PUBLIC LAW 93-360**
>
> The professional employee is:
> (a) any employee engaged in work (i) predominantly intellectual and varied in character as opposed to routine mental, manual, mechanical, or physical work; (ii) involving the consistent exercise of discretion and judgment in its performance; (iii) of such a character that the output produced or the result accomplished cannot be standardized in relation to a given period of time; (iv) requiring knowledge of an advanced type in a field of science or learning customarily acquired by a prolonged course of specialized intellectual instruction and study in an institution of higher learning or a hospital, as distinguished from a general academic education or from an apprenticeship or from training in the performance of routine mental, manual, or physical processes; or (b) any employee, who (i) has completed the courses of specialized intellectual instruction and study described in clause (iv) of paragraph (a), and (ii) is performing related work under the supervision of a professional person to qualify himself to become a professional employee as defined in paragraph (a).[6]

National registration and certification do not provide a legal basis for practicing respiratory care by itself. The legal basis for practicing a profession is left to the regulation of individual states.[7] States generally adopt licensing laws, known as practice acts, to carry out this regulatory process. An administrative or regulatory agency then adopts more specific requirements to be followed to grant a state license to individual practitioners.

There is often confusion about the actual meaning of the terms "licensure," "certification," and "registration." A major reason for the confusion is that the terms are not always used correctly. For example, the title Registered Nurse, implying registration, is usually reserved for use by nurses who are licensed by the state. This "registered" title is used although all 50 states have strong nurse practice acts which are actually licensing acts. Yet, the term "registration," when used properly, denotes the weakest form of professional regulation. This paradox apparently exists in nursing because the first nurse's "licensing act" in 1903 was in fact a registration act. It was not mandatory for the practice of nursing.[8]

The most formal and strongest form of professional regulation is licensure. Licenses are issued by a designated state agency under a law generally referred to for health care workers as a practice act. A licensed professional must meet education and other legal requirements as defined by the practice act and which may be further specified in the regulations adopted under the act. The practice act usually prohibits unlicensed individuals from practicing the regulated profession.[9]

By definition, the second strongest form of professional regulation is certification. However, in practice, this may not be the case. Certification implies that the professional has demonstrated in some manner, usually by examination, a specified level of competency. Certification is generally voluntary and without legal consequences for those who do not seek certification. Thus, a noncertified professional may be able to practice the same profession as a certified professional without any fear of legal consequences from a credentialing standpoint.[10] However, all practitioners are cautioned to clearly determine and comply with the legal requirements for practice in their individual states.

The word "registration" is derived from "registry." It implies that a list or registry is maintained of professionals. The purpose is usually to inform the public or prospective employers that the registered individual has met certain requirements to be placed on the list. Individuals who have not met the specified requirements and have not registered cannot refer to themselves as registered professionals. Registration does not carry legal prohibitions that prevent nonregistered individuals from practicing the specified profession.[10] When registration is required by state law, it is called title protection.

## State Respiratory Care Practice Acts

The American Association for Respiratory Care, the major national professional organization for respiratory care practitioners, has long had as one of its objectives state licensure for its members. To date, 37 states and Puerto Rico have adopted legislation that establishes some form of regulation for respiratory care practitioners. There is ongoing, intense activity in the majority of the remaining states to pass legislation for the regulation of respiratory care practitioners within their borders.

Licensure serves many functions. The primary function of licensure is to define who can and cannot practice a given profession. In theory, the individual licensee and the governmental entity granting the license, usually the state, have a single purpose for licensure. That purpose is to provide for public safety. However, in reality, there may be additional purposes for licensure. For example, from the individual practitioner's standpoint, besides providing public safety, licensure is generally seen as a measure of professionalism and of the status of a profession.

The regulation of the practice of respiratory care currently in effect takes one of two forms: title protection and licensing. Nine states currently have title protection statutes (Box 2–3), whereas 28 states and Puerto Rico have practice acts that constitutes licensing. Title protection acts regulate who may or may not use a title that identifies the user as a respiratory care practitioner. The assumption is that the public will be protected since it will be easy to identify those practitioners entitled to call themselves respiratory care practitioners. The actual title may vary from state to state. The drawback with title protection statutes is that they do not prohibit the practice of respiratory care by any individuals as long as they do not refer to themselves as respiratory care practitioners. Title protection statutes are often adopted in those states where the political climate makes it difficult or impossible to pass a more restrictive licensure statute.

> **Box 2-3. STATES WITH TITLE PROTECTION STATUTES FOR RESPIRATORY CARE PRACTITIONERS**
>
> Connecticut
> Indiana
> Kansas
> Minnesota
> Pennsylvania
> South Carolina
> Virginia
> Washington
> Missouri

In states with practice acts (Box 2-4), only those individuals who are licensed may practice respiratory care. Licensure also provides title protection; however, it goes significantly further toward ensuring public safety since it actually prohibits unlicensed individuals from practicing.

All states with either title protection or practice acts currently use the credentialing process already established by the NBRC. However, it should be noted, that merely possessing registration or certification from the NBRC does not constitute the legal authority to practice. The practitioner must still apply to the appropriate state agency and comply with their requirements before the legal authority to practice, a state license, will be granted.

## General Components of Respiratory Care Practice Acts

Respiratory care practice acts vary from state to state. However, there are generally some standard components included in most practice acts. Most practice acts consist of two parts. The first part consists of the statute that was passed by the state's legislative body and signed by the governor. The second part consists of the rules developed by the board or council appointed to administer the statute. The statute will be broad in scope and can be changed only by legislation. The rules are more definitive and can be changed by the board or council as long as the changes are within the limits established by the statute. It is extremely important for respiratory care practitioners to be knowledgeable about the entire practice act of their state.

Following is a list of some of the standard components of statutes that regulate respiratory care along with an explanation of the purpose of each component.

*Title* This part states the legal title of the statute.

*Purpose, Intent, and Application* In this part the need for the statute is set forth. Language will usually be included that refers to providing for public health and safety. The target profession will also be identified.

### Box 2-4. STATES WITH RESPIRATORY CARE PRACTICE ACTS (LICENSURE)*

Arizona
Arkansas
California
Florida
Georgia
Idaho
Iowa
Kentucky
Louisiana
Maine
Maryland
Massachusetts
Mississippi
Montana
Nebraska
New Hampshire
New Jersey
New Mexico
New York
North Dakota
Ohio
Oregon
Rhode Island
South Dakota
Tennessee
Texas
Utah
Wisconsin

*Puerto Rico also has a practice act.

*Definitions* This part defines the key terms included in the statute. Generally, a definition of respiratory care will also be included.

*Administering Authority* This part will give the authority for establishing the board, council, or agency that will administer the practice act. Composition of the board or council, terms of service, duties, and authority of the body will also be defined.

*Eligibility for Licensing* This part defines the qualifications that prospective licensees must meet. Qualifications are generally defined in terms of age, education, and credentialing from other sources. General requirements for most states include attainment of the age of 18, possession of a high school diploma, and certification or registration from the NBRC. Exemptions, if any, from these requirements are also usually included in this part. For example, most statutes contain a "grandfather clause" that allows those practicing at the time the statute is adopted to be licensed if they have practiced for a specified period of time, although they do not meet the current educational qualifications.

*Licensing Process*   There may be several parts dealing with licensing. The purpose is to establish the actual process that the prospective licensee must follow in order to obtain the license. Sections may be included addressing licensing by examination for the new graduate and by endorsement for practitioners holding a credential from another agency, for example, an NBRC-registered respiratory therapist. Additional sections falling under this general topic will deal with the administrative process of the use of titles, the license renewal process, continuing education, and reactivation of inactive licenses.

*Fees*   This part will establish the fees for services such as examinations, initial licensing, and licensing renewal. A flat fee may be established or a range of fees may be listed with the specific fee to be decided by the board or council.

*Disciplinary Grounds and Actions*   This part defines those acts or failures to act that constitute grounds for disciplinary actions. The range of penalties that may be imposed also will be defined. As stated earlier, practice acts vary considerably from state to state.

The components listed here are neither all-inclusive or all-exclusive. It is the responsibility of each respiratory care practitioner to be aware of the contents of the practice act in the local state of employment.

## POTENTIAL LIABILITY IN RESPIRATORY CARE PRACTICE

The respiratory care practitioner has a legal responsibility to perform duties in a competent manner. Failure to do so will result in a situation where the practitioner must assume professional liability for his or her actions.

### Professional Liability

There are several situations in which respiratory care practitioners may find themselves facing professional liability. The type of liability will depend on the type of action the practitioner took or failed to take. Many of these actions fall under what is classified as tort law. A *tort* is a civil wrongdoing committed toward someone that results in harm or injury.[11] A discussion follows of some of the torts that practitioners may face.

When a practitioner intentionally engages in noncriminal behavior prohibited by law and injury or harm occurs to the patient, it is called an *intentional* tort. Since one of the characteristics of intentional torts is that the practitioner intended to commit the act, intentional torts are more serious than those torts which do not require proof of intent, such as negligence. The classic example of an intentional tort is assault and battery. It should be noted that both assault and battery can be personal torts as well as criminal offenses. Although we might seldom think of assault or battery as issues for practitioners, battery, in particular, can easily occur between practitioners and patients. Assault is defined as an action that places someone in fear of personal injury. The best example of an assault is a threat, accompanied by a physical manifestation, for example, clenched fists, to do bodily harm to someone.

From a criminal standpoint, battery is thought of as actually carrying out a threat to do bodily harm. In reality, battery can be as simple as touching someone without his or her consent. Thus, although unlikely in most cases, a practitioner could be accused of battery if there is a failure to obtain permission from a patient to perform a given procedure. When patients are hospitalized, the potential of a practitioner being accused of battery drops considerably since by presenting themselves for treatment, patients give implied consent for procedures that are considered ordinary for the condition being treated. Some specific procedures may require that the patient sign a permission form, although most procedures performed by respiratory care practitioners will not have specific permissions forms. In all cases, however, it is important to explain to the patient the procedure to be performed and pay close attention to any efforts the patient makes to refuse the procedure or to withdraw consent. Regardless of the legal considerations, it is simply good practice for practitioners to explain all procedures to patients even if there is reason to believe that the patient is incapable of understanding. Other intentional torts that are particularly relevant to respiratory care practitioners include invasion of privacy and defamation. For practitioners, these torts can be closely related.

Invasion of privacy is likely to become an issue when a practitioner purposely seeks information about a patient that the practitioner does not need to know in order to perform his or her duties. If that information is then used in a manner that is harmful to the patient, another tort, defamation of character, may be present. Even if the information is necessary for the performance of the practitioner's duties, publicly revealing information about a private individual constitutes invasion of privacy. Additionally, this would be a violation of patient-practitioner confidentiality, one of the ethical issues that will be dealt with in later in this book.

Defamation of character may take one of two forms: libel or slander. Libel refers to a written statement, and slander refers to a spoken statement. Both statements must be untrue and must be seen or heard by a third party. The practitioner should note, however, that the truthfulness of the statement is not an absolute protection since there could still be an issue of invasion of privacy or violation of confidentiality laws or rules.

A second type of tort that could arise for a practitioner is negligence. Simply speaking, negligence is the failure of a professional to perform a duty in a competent manner. It should be noted that the standard of competence may be defined differently in different locales. When considering negligence claims, terms such as "ordinary," "gross," "contributory," and "comparative" may be used. Using these terms to define the extent and to allocate damages in negligence cases is a complex process and is best left to legal counsel.

In evaluating negligence claims, several factors must be identifiable. First, the practitioner must clearly have had a duty to perform. Second, it must be clear that the practitioner failed to perform at an acceptable level of competence. Third, it must be clear that the failure of the practitioner to perform at the acceptable level was the direct cause of damages suffered by the patient. When these factors are present, the patient may be awarded monetary damages for his or her injury.

*Professional malpractice* is negligence in which it is alleged that a professional has failed to provide the care expected of that type of professional and that the substandard care resulted in harm to someone. Examples of professional malpractice that respiratory care practitioners may find themselves involved in include:

**Performing Procedures Beyond the Scope of One's Training and Education**
Nothing, other than hospital policy, prevents a practitioner with 20 years of service in adult critical care from working in a neonatal intensive care unit. Based on actual experience, however, it is unlikely that such a practitioner would be competent with newborns. If such a practitioner were to provide neonatal critical care and cause harm to a patient, such action would likely provide the basis for a professional malpractice claim.

**Attempting to Treat Too Many Patients Simultaneously, Resulting in Harm to One or More Patients**   Given the existing staffing shortages in some institutions, it might appear admirable to provide care to all patients even if the quality of care suffers. Admittedly, the resolution to this situation is complex. However, the practitioner needs to be aware that providing substandard care, under any circumstances, can result in a malpractice claim.

The above examples of professional malpractice are not meant to be exhaustive. The intent of the examples is to raise the awareness of practitioners as to the type of situations that could give rise to a claim of professional malpractice. It is important that the practitioner notes that professional malpractice does not require any intent to cause harm but that harm must occur in order for malpractice to exist.

An important doctrine of negligence that practitioners should be aware of is *res ipsa loquitur,* "the thing speaks for itself." This doctrine is invoked when negligence is obvious. For example, if an improperly assembled ventilator circuit causes a patient to experience severe hypoxia, it may be said that "the thing (the improperly assembled circuit) speaks for itself."

## Malpractice Prevention

Prevention is the best treatment for professional malpractice, and there are three options available. If the practitioner maintains an appropriate standard of care, follows policies and procedures, adheres to quality assurance standards, and complies with any risk management recommendations, the incidences of professional malpractice would be greatly reduced. Standard of care refers to care that is reasonable and ordinary for the professional and the condition. It is the type of care that any other practitioner would be expected to offer under the same circumstances in that community. For example, if an average adult patient requires a 7.5-mm endotracheal tube for intubation, a practitioner would be going outside the standard of care if an attempt was made to insert a 10.0-mm tube without a clear and logical reason for selecting the larger tube. Policies and procedures provide guidelines for standards of care. Every workplace should have updated policies and procedures for all duties or tasks that are to be performed. There should also be a policy and procedures to cover unexpected duties or tasks. These documents provide protection to both the practitioner and the institution in that they standardize the type and quality of care to be delivered.

Quality assurance is a relatively new procedure adopted by health care institutions. The focus of quality assurance is to detect flaws in procedures that result in low-quality care. These flaws are then corrected to ensure the delivery of high-quality care to patients. Most institutions initially adopted quality assurance programs as a method of increasing efficiency and reducing cost. Since then, the Joint Committee on Accreditation of Healthcare Organizations (JCAHO) has adopted quality assurance standards to be used by all accredited institutions. An effective quality assurance program will significantly reduce incidents of malpractice.

Risk management is a formalized process of systematically evaluating the risks faced by the department and the institution. If the risk is too great, steps will be taken to decrease it. Large institutions have professional risk managers on staff to facilitate this process.

## Malpractice Protection

When the various malpractice preventive measures fail, it is important to have financial protection against malpractice losses. This protection comes in the form of professional liability insurance. If the respiratory care practitioner is employed by an institution, he or she will be covered by the institution's liability insurance as long as the duties performed are within the limits of the job description.

Respiratory care practitioners who practice independently through contract services may need to purchase individual liability insurance. The cost is relatively inexpensive compared to the cost to institutions and primary practitioners like physicians. The issue of whether all practitioners should maintain liability insurance is widely debated. Each practitioner must weigh the pros and cons and decide on the best avenue to take.

## APPLIED EXERCISES

1. Review the legislative actions from your state's most recent session and determine which, if any, laws were passed that will have a clear and direct impact on the health care industry.
2. Locate at least two legal decisions handed down by the courts in the past 3 years that may potentially have a direct impact on the practice of respiratory care.

3. Take one of the following positions: (A) Respiratory care practitioners are professionals. (B) Respiratory care practitioners are not professionals. Use the definition of professionals presented in this chapter to defend your position.

## STUDY QUESTIONS

1. The roots of the American legal system are found in the common law of what country? What are some of the elements from that system that are included in the American legal system?

2. What are the two divisions of statutory law?

3. Briefly discuss the role of law in providing guidelines for behavior in our society.

4. Briefly discuss the relationship seen by the reader, if any, between societal values, ethics, and the law.

5. Laws made by what bodies are most likely to impact the respiratory care practitioner? Briefly explain why.

6. Distinguish between the following levels of credentials: registration, certification, and licensure. Briefly discuss the difference between how they are used and the actual legal definitions of each.

7. *Given an example of* res ipsa loquitur.

8. *Distinguish between "the greater weight of the evidence" and "beyond a reasonable doubt."*

9. *What is the meaning of "title protection"?*

10. *Briefly describe the role of the board or council in state charged with the regulation of the practice of respiratory care.*

## REFERENCES

1. Lewis, MA, and Warden, CD: Law and Ethics in the Medical Office, ed 2. FA Davis, Philadelphia, 1988, p 33.
2. Biggs, D: How to Avoid Lawyers. Garland, New York, 1985.
3. Flight, MR: Law, Liability, and Ethics. Delmar, Albany, NY, 1988.
4. Eicher, J: State credentialing update. AARC Times, March 1994.
5. Labor Management Relations Act (1947) as amended by Public Laws 86-257 (1959) and 93-360 (1974), sec ?
6. Annas, G, et al: The Rights of Doctors, Nurses and Allied Health Professionals. Ballinger, Cambridge, MA, 1981, p 3.
7. Ibid, p 5.
8. Ibid. p 45.
9. Ibid, p 44.
10. Ibid, p 369.
11. Gifis, SH: Law Dictionary. Barron's, New York, 1975.

# CHAPTER 3

# *Ethics and Health Care*

**Definitions of Ethics**
**The Foundation of Ethical Thinking**
Ethical Principles
Ethical Theories
**Health, Disease, and Ethics**
**Who Is Entitled to Health Care?**
**Health Care Versus Disease Care**
**The Role of Ethics in Health Care**

## DEFINITIONS OF ETHICS

Ethics is a frequently discussed concept among health care professionals. Unfortunately, there is limited understanding as to the actual meaning of "health care ethics." One reason is that the term is difficult to define precisely. The Greek *ethos,* from which the word "ethics" is derived, is defined as "custom or practice, a characteristic manner of acting, a more or less constant mode of behavior in the deliberate actions of men."[1] "Customs or practices" can obviously vary considerably from time to time and from place to place. The phrase "characteristic manner of acting" raises the question: to whom is the manner of acting characteristic? One conclusion that can be drawn from these two phrases is that the definition of ethics must be considered relative to the time, place, and setting involved. Once the time, place, and setting are established, then we may focus on the basic definition of ethics as the study of right and wrong.[2] Of course, this definition still brings to mind the questions: what is right, what is wrong, and who decides? The answer to the first two questions is constantly being redefined, depending on the time, place, and setting. The answer to the third question lies in the concept of universal principles as adopted by a society.

Certain universal principles are accepted by the majority of our society, and among them are generally accepted beliefs of right and wrong. In fact, Dyck[3] defined ethics as an expression of the feelings of the majority. On the other hand, Findley[4] provides a more formal definition of ethics, which states that ethics is the systematic study of voluntary acts which affect the welfare of living creatures.

Regardless of the definition, most of us agree that to be ethical means to behave at the highest level of rightness for the greatest good; to be ethical means that one's actions are beyond reproach. A discussion on the definition of ethics would not be complete without describing some of the subdivisions of ethics. One way of subdividing ethics is to separate it into two categories called normative and nonnormative. *Normative ethics* deals with prescriptive processes, whereas *nonnormative ethics* deals with what people actually believe and do (descriptive) and with the language, reasoning, and logic of ethics (meta-ethics). This text discusses normative ethics only.

Normative ethics can be classified by the type of situation involved, for example, professional ethics, general ethics, bioethics, or business ethics. This text will focus on professional ethics and bioethics. *Professional ethics* refers to a standard of behavior adopted by a professional group. *Bioethics* deals specifically with general ethics as it applies to medicine.

## THE FOUNDATION OF ETHICAL THINKING

One way to get a clearer picture of the meaning of ethics is to look at some of the concepts that either form the foundation for ethics or at least impact our individual ethical thinking. At least four concepts should be considered: personal beliefs, personal attitudes, personal values, and personal morals. Concepts that may form the foundation for an individual's ethical thinking are:
1. Ethical orientation
2. Moral philosophy
3. Personal value system
4. Attitudinal orientation
5. Personal belief system

Each of these items builds on the item below it, integrating the components until finally an ethical orientation is developed. Theoretically, the ethical orientation is at a higher level of consciousness than its component parts; however, this is not necessarily the case since different individuals give varying weights to the component parts.

In order to further understand the meaning of ethics, it may be helpful if we define the component parts from which our ethical orientation is derived. Our personal belief system is based on personal convictions that we develop from various life experiences. It is not an objective system and may not work in our best interest. However, it is what we believe, and it forms the basis for our opinions.

The application of our opinions forms our attitudinal orientation; that is, we behave as we believe. When we are so strongly committed to our attitudes that we are unwilling to change or modify them when given conflicting information, we have then given the attitudes the status of being part of our personal principles. These principles make up our personal value system.

**Table 3–1.** KOHLBERG'S STAGES IN THE DEVELOPMENT OF MORAL THINKING

| STAGE | OUTCOME |
|---|---|
| 1 | We focus on obedience and punishment. |
| 2 | We concentrate on making a "good deal." |
| 3 | We emphasize the importance of conforming to the expectations of those who are close to us. |
| 4 | We stress laws, social duties, and conscience. |
| 5 | We recognize that most values and rights are relative, but some, such as life and liberty, should be upheld in any society. |
| 6 | We focus exclusively on universal moral principles. |

Our personal values determine the moral orientation that we exhibit. Morals define what we consider to be right. They are not static; that is, they can and do change. When society as a group shares a set of morals, then these morals may become universal principles and gain status as ethically "correct." In some cases, they may be adopted as law. Since ethical behavior is, in part, an expression of our moral thinking, it is important to understand how our moral thinking is developed as our beliefs and values are incorporated into our morals. Psychologist Lawrence Kohlberg developed a series of predictable stages that many of us go through as we develop our moral thinking. These stages are summarized in Table 3–1.[5]

Kohlberg's stages of moral development are the result of a 20-year longitudinal study designed to answer questions on the process of moral development. Although the results of his study have been widely accepted, they have also been widely debated. One of the major criticisms directed toward Kohlberg was that all the subjects in the study were American men. Carol Gilligan, in her 1982 book, *In a Different Voice,* challenged Kohlberg's study and criticized its failure to deal with the female viewpoint. She maintains that the moral development process of women is different from that of men.[6]

If you have drawn the conclusion from our discussion so far that one's ethical orientation is a dynamic rather than a static process, you are absolutely correct. However, do not take that conclusion to mean that ethical orientation is a totally unstable concept. Neither individual nor societal ethical orientations change very rapidly.

Stability is maintained because society's ethical orientation is greater than the sum of its parts; that is, it is greater than each individual's ethical orientation. This makes it difficult, although not impossible, for an individual to rapidly change personal views on ethical behavior. Therefore, at any given point in time, there is a strong likelihood that the ethical orientation of individuals will be in keeping with the universal principles accepted by society.

## Ethical Principles

Traditionally, there were 12 generally accepted universal ethical principles, elements, or, as they are sometimes called, standards[7]:

- Autonomy
- Beneficence
- Confidentiality
- Fidelity
- Justice
- Nonmaleficence
- Paternalism
- Quality of life
- Reparation
- Sanctity of life
- Utilitarianism
- Veracity

Contemporary ethicists, arguing that the traditional ethical principles created impossible dilemmas, have narrowed the number to approximately six[8]:

- Autonomy
- Veracity
- Beneficence
- Freedom
- Privacy
- Fidelity

The extent to which these principles are accepted and the relative importance afforded each principle are based on the beliefs, values, and morals of the individual. Both the traditional and contemporary principles are discussed in detail in Chapter 5.

## Ethical Theories

In addition to ethical principles, there are also several ethical theories. The relationship between ethical principles and theories is not always clear. In fact, some ethicists have noted conflict between the principles and theories.[9] Despite this seeming conflict, ethical principles and theories are incorporated into most ethical decision-making models. There are two major ethical theories, deontological and utilitarian.

The *deontological* ethical theory grew out of the eighteenth-century philosophy advanced by Immanuel Kant; the theory emphasizes duties, rights, and responsibilities. The *utilitarian* theory is one of a group of theories called the teleological theories; the utilitarian theory is usually associated with eighteenth-century philosopher Jeremy Bentham and nineteenth-century philosopher John Stuart Mill. It focuses on the "utility" or usefulness of an action. (Both theories will be discussed in greater detail in Chapter 6.)

## HEALTH, DISEASE, AND ETHICS

In the delivery of health care services one is confronted by many ethical issues. Some of the issues are more global in nature, whereas others are practical, everyday concerns. Box 3–1 lists some of the more common practical concerns. The items were

> **Box 3–1. ETHICAL ISSUES OF A PRACTICAL NATURE IN HEALTH CARE**
>
> 1. Do not resuscitate (DNR) orders
> 2. Confidentiality of patient's records
> 3. Termination of life support equipment
> 4. Inadequate staffing for safe care of patients
> 5. Inability of patients to pay for services
> 6. Conflict between patients and family members
> 7. Incompetence on the part of fellow practitioners
> 8. Impaired performance by fellow practitioners
> 9. Allocation of resources
> 10. Equal treatment (justice) for all patients

obtained from a survey of allied health instructors who are also allied health professionals. You may think of other items to add to this list. Certainly, within a few years of working as a health professional, you will be able to add some issues that are unique to your institution or work setting.

It should be noted that most of the items in Box 3–1 have the potential for legal complications, but most of them are not dealt with from a legal standpoint. The celebrated legal cases in connection with the delivery of health care services represent only a few of the many ethical dilemmas health care practitioners handle on a daily basis.

Health, disease, and ethics are integrally entwined. Any attempt to resolve issues associated with the far-from-exclusive list of issues identified in Box 3–1 immediately raises ethical considerations. A sampling of these considerations is offered below in order to prepare the reader for the type of ethical issues and questions that we deal with later in this text.

*Do not resuscitate orders*
1. Is the patient terminal?
2. Is the patient's quality of life unbearable?
3. How much care should the patient be given?

*Confidentiality of patient's records*
1. Should all records be confidential under all circumstances?
2. Who has a right to know what's in a patient's records?
3. When is the public's right to know greater than the patient's right to confidentiality?

*Termination of life support equipment*
1. What exactly is life support?
2. Who decides when and how to terminate life support?

3. What if the patient does not die when life support is terminated?
4. Can the money spent on hopeless life support be better spent on promoting health?

*Inadequate staffing for safe patient care*
1. How can staffing ratios be determined?
2. Should staffing be for minimum, optimal, or maximum care?
3. Is staffing related more to numbers of personnel or to skill of personnel?

*Inability of patients to pay for services*
1. Should care be given regardless of ability to pay?
2. Who pays when patients cannot pay?
3. Should paying patients and nonpaying patients receive the same care?

*Conflict between patient and family*
1. Who knows best, the patient or the family?
2. What if the patient is incompetent?
3. What if the family has unknown motives?

*Incompetence on the part of fellow practitioners*
1. How can incompetence be recognized and defined?
2. Whose responsibility is it to report incompetence?
3. To whom should incompetence be reported?

*Impaired performance by fellow practitioners*
1. How can impairment be recognized and defined?
2. How much impairment is too much?
3. Should the practitioner be given an opportunity to recognize and deal with his/her own impairment? To whom should impairment be reported?

*Allocation of resources*
1. Should available funds be spent for disease care or preventive health care?
2. Should funds be spent on basic care for many or advanced care for a few?
3. How should funds for research be allocated?

*Equal treatment (justice) for all patients*
1. Should patients with preventable diseases be treated the same as patients with diseases they could not prevent?
2. Which is more important, providing care to patients or decreasing the risk to the care giver?
3. Should the age, race, gender, or national origin impact the level of care?
4. Who is entitled to health care?

The questions raised here are complex, and the answers will not be any less complex. Health professionals, on any level, cannot be expected to provide completely satisfactory answers to all these questions. The aim of this book is simply to provide a framework within which respiratory care practitioners can ethically consider each of these questions as well as the many other questions that may arise while dealing with the challenges of promoting health and eliminating disease.

## WHO IS ENTITLED TO HEALTH CARE?

One of the questions raised in the previous section deserves some special attention at this point since it is at the root of many contemporary discussions of ethics and health care. This question centers on the availability of resources for providing health care: When resources are limited, who is entitled to them? No attempt will be made to provide a definitive answer to this question in this text; the purpose here is merely to call attention to the ethical dilemma created by our current limited health care resources. However, the question can be answered in part by utilizing the ethical decision-making processes discussed in Chapter 4, the ethical theories in Chapter 6, and the ethical principles discussed in Chapter 4.

At this point in considering the question of who is entitled to health care, it may be useful to discuss two additional concepts. The first concept deals with whether health care is a right or a privilege. The second concept deals with the definition of health care in terms of minimum or maximum care. Using the four components of these two concepts, four position statements can be developed. As you will see in the discussion on ethical principles, each of these positions can be supported or opposed by one or more of the ethical principles. The relative importance, or weight, assigned to the principles is used by individuals to decide whether they support or oppose the positions expressed in the statements.

*Minimum Health Care Is a Right to Which Everyone Is Entitled*   Proponents of this position maintain that resources should be made available to provide basic care for everyone. This position usually means that highly expensive care such as long-term life support and high-risk surgical procedures such as transplants would be eliminated. Preventive health care would also be emphasized.

*Maximum Health Care Is a Right to Which Everyone Is Entitled*   Proponents of this position maintain that all known therapy, procedures, and equipment should be available to everyone. Cost should not be a factor. It would be the joint responsibility of the people and government to ensure that the needed resources are funded.

*Minimum Health Care Is a Privilege to Which Some People Are Entitled*   Proponents of this position maintain that even minimum health care is a privilege. It would be up to each individual to develop his or her own resources to pay for this minimum care. If a person were unable to do so, then health care would be unavailable.

*Maximum Health Care Is a Privilege to Which Some People Are Entitled*   Proponents of this position generally state that they are in favor of health care for everyone. However, they believe that some resources must be allocated for expensive advanced therapy, procedures, and equipment. Their reasoning is based in part on the argument that medical advances, which benefit everyone, are made only when there is a continuous effort to use new technology to the maximum. Ironically, those who can afford to pay for expensive care are not the only people to benefit from this position since a large portion of advanced care is offered in teaching hospitals where many of the patient population are indigent.

At first glance, it may appear to be easy to decide which of the above positions is the right one. In reality, none of the positions is as simple as it may appear. In fact, there may be a clear difference between a stated position and the reality that occurs when it is applied. As indicated earlier, the purpose of our discussion here is not to tell the student which position to take. The purpose of this discussion is to raise the student's awareness of the dilemmas one may be confronted with when applying ethical principles and theories.

## HEALTH CARE VERSUS DISEASE CARE

Health care in America is big business, with rapidly increasing costs and complexities. When Medicare was introduced in 1965, the cost of delivering health services was a mere $42 billion. By 1987, the bill was more than $500 billion. Although the final cost for 1995 is not yet available, it is expected that the cost will exceed a trillion dollars. If this projection is realized, the cost of Medicare will represent 14 percent of our gross national product. With more than 8.5 million individuals employed in health care services, the opportunities for ethical dilemmas are numerous.

The goals set for a nation's health care system contribute to the development of ethical dilemmas. The focus of the American health care system is largely "disease care"; that is, care is centers on correcting pathological processes rather than preventing disease in the first place. Although there has been some effort to reallocate resources toward prevention, the system continues to care for patients primarily after they have contracted a disease and are very sick. The rationale for focusing on disease care as opposed to preventive health care is not clear. It might be argued that both disease and health care are one and the same. Such an argument would assume that health and disease are on opposite ends of the same continuum. Although there is some prima facie evidence for such an argument, being disease-free is not necessarily the same as being healthy. This is not a new debate, and it is likely to become more intense in the coming years as the cost of providing care to the sick continues to increase exponentially. In the final analysis, it may be simply that our society places a greater value on being disease-free than on being healthy.

From an application standpoint, the "disease care" focus presents several ethical dilemmas that would be lessened under a health care model that focused appropriately on prevention as well as on correction of pathological processes. First, preventive health care is generally less expensive than corrective health care. Second, preventive health care can be practiced in a less intense environment which allows for a more systematic approach to ethical decision making. Third, the delivery of disease care is complicated by our society's obsession with longevity and immortality. This obsession adds an emotional component to the process that intensifies any ethical dilemma that might arise. Finally, for the health care practitioner, whether we call our system "health care" or "disease care" may be less important than whether we deliver quality care in keeping with ethical codes of conduct.

## THE ROLE OF ETHICS IN HEALTH CARE

Ethics serves many roles. A major role is to serve as a tool for decision making when a person or institution is faced with an ethical dilemma. Probably the highest calling of ethics is to serve as a societal standard of behavior that brings some level of reason and stability to our actions. Ethics can also be used as a personal coping mechanism to assist individuals in understanding and coping with ethical dilemmas in which they may be involved. As a decision-making tool, the study of ethics provides several model frameworks that can used by decision makers. By definition, an ethical dilemma requires one to choose between two equally desirable or undesirable choices. The frameworks are useful because they allow the decision maker to look at the relative importance of the component parts rather than to focus on the overall dilemma.

Although a decision made by two different people may differ, the process ensures that, as a whole, similar people will make similar decisions. Since similar people tend to make similar ethical decisions, the stability of our society is enhanced. In addition to the importance of making ethical decisions, understanding and acceptance is important for those who are involved in or affected by the decisions. Respiratory care practitioners must not only participate in numerous ethical decisions but must also deal with the outcome of numerous decisions over which they have no control. A thorough understanding of ethics will assist in this process. Thus, the study of ethics not only provides a guide for behaving but also serves as an adjunct to understanding the behavior of others.

## APPLIED EXERCISES

1. Talk to several health care professionals, and ask them to describe ethical dilemmas that occur regularly in the health care setting. If you are in clinical training, you should have easy access to professionals in your major field of study; if not, ask several of your instructors for help. Make a list of these ethical dilemmas for future use.
2. Expand the discussion of health care versus disease care by seeking to define these terms as precisely as possible. Research the current literature on these topics and support your definitions with the points of view raised by others.

## STUDY QUESTIONS

1. What is a very basic definition of ethics? What are some of the problems with a short simplistic definition of such a complex term?

2. What is a more formal definition of ethics? Discuss the practical application of such a definition.

3. What is the basis of our personal belief system?

4. What is the basis of our attitudinal orientation?

5. When our attitudinal orientation is strong enough to withstand challenges, what status do our attitudes assume?

6. What is the basis for our personal value system?

7. In which stage did Kohlberg first mention the concept of values?

8. What type of ethics deals with what people actually believe and do?

9. What type of ethics deals specifically with general ethics as applied to medicine?

## REFERENCES

1. Davis, AJ, and Aroskar, MA: Ethical Dilemmas and Nursing Practice. Appleton-Century-Crofts, New York, 1978, p 1.
2. Lewis, MA, and Warden, CD: Law and Ethics in the Medical Office, ed 2. FA Davis, Philadelphia, 1988, p 33.
3. Dyck, A: On Human Care: An Introduction to Ethics. Parthenon Press, Nashville, TN, 1977.
4. Findley, JN: Introductory Readings in Ethics. Prentice Hall, Englewood Cliffs, NJ, 1974.
5. Lickona, T (Ed): Moral Development and Behavior: Theory, Research and Social Issues. Holt, Rinehart and Winston, New York, 1976, pp 34–35.
6. Gilligan, C: In a Different Voice. Harvard University Press, Cambridge, MA, 1982.
7. Beauchamp, TL, and Childress, JE: Principles of Biomedical Ethics, ed 2. Oxford University Press, New York, 1983.
8. Husted, GL, and Husted, JH: Ethical Decision Making in Nursing. Mosby Year Book, St Louis, 1991, p 40.
9. Ibid, p 60.

# CHAPTER 4

# *The Ethical Decision-Making Process*

**The Basis of Ethical Decisions**
**Who Makes Ethical Decisions?**
Ethical Autonomy
**Participating in Ethical Decision Making**
Ethics Committees
Decision Making as a Process
The Individual Decision-Making Process

## THE BASIS OF ETHICAL DECISIONS

It is easy to visualize ethical decision making as an abstract process, far removed from the duties and responsibilities of the typical workday. Even though most health care practitioners are guided by a code of ethics that has been adopted by their professional organization, the tendency still exists to view ethical decision making as an abstract process. This is unfortunate since numerous ethical decisions are made routinely by the average health care practitioner on a daily basis.

Since ethical decision making is often seen as an abstract process, most health care practitioners are unprepared for making ethical decisions on a routine basis. As a result, they often experience considerable distress when expected to participate in such grave decisions. Often, the solution is to "pass the buck" to someone else or to simply refuse to become involved. Neither solution is acceptable. Instead, we must find ways of preparing professionals for such decisions. First, all health care practitioners should receive in-depth instruction in professional health care ethics as part of their professional education. Second, all health care practitioners must be made aware of the vital role they play in ethical decision making. They cannot be allowed to assume that the responsibility for such decisions belongs to someone else. As a member of a health care profession and as a member of society at large, every health care practitioner has an obligation to contribute to ethical decision making.

There is a generally accepted principle that in order to make good and informed ethical decisions, the decision maker must be able to meet three requirements. He or she must be able to (1) understand the options presented by the different alternatives, (2) know the risks and potential consequences of each of the different alternatives, and (3) freely choose the best of the alternatives. If any of these requirements is not present, the decision maker's ability to make an ethical decision is compromised.[1]

If the ethical decision maker can meet the three requirements listed above, it is then vital that one of the models of ethical analysis be utilized to finalize the decision. Remember, since the decision may have to be made quickly, the decision maker must have a clear understanding of the model prior to the time a decision is needed. Three models for making ethical decisions are presented in Chapter 7.

It should also be noted here that the ethical decision maker brings to the process all of his or her life experiences. These life experiences include personal and professional codes of ethics. Also included are the decision maker's thoughts and experiences on personal beliefs, values, and morals. The decision maker may never have heard of an ethical principle or theory, but in essence he or she will have formulated such a working principle or theory utilizing personal thought processes. These working formulations will impact the decision-making process. This is also true for formal theories such as the theory of moral development presented by Lawrence Kohlberg that was later challenged by Carol Gilligan. For, if these theories are valid, one does not have to be aware of them before being affected by them. Health care workers, in particular, are likely to have opinions regarding health and disease and the rights and privileges involved with health care, as well as the concept of delivering minimum versus maximum care. All of their opinions will impact the decision-making process.

## WHO MAKES ETHICAL DECISIONS?

Every individual makes ethical decisions at some time. Health care practitioners at all levels are no exception. Regardless of the job responsibilities of a particular worker, ethical decisions must be made in a variety of situations. Any time you make a decision that impacts the well-being or welfare of another person, you have engaged in ethical decision making.

Acceptance of the responsibility for ethical decision making by health care practitioners is extremely important because of the nature of our work. The delivery of our services tends to have a direct, and in many cases an immediate, impact on the lives of our patients and clients. Furthermore, patients depend on our expertise for the maintenance of their health and well-being. Finally, unlike other nonmedical situations where an individual may have recourse to damages because of injury, the damage caused by a health care practitioner may be irreversible. Therefore, while the practitioner cannot ensure that all treatments will have the desired outcome, it is essential that they not be guilty of neglecting their ethical responsibility.

The importance of everyone being involved in the ethical decision-making process has been emphasized by Zbigniew Bankowski, Secretary-General, Council for International Organizations of Medical Sciences in Geneva, Switzerland. He states that the extent to which we are willing to make ethical decisions is a measure of our understanding of what it means to be human.[2]

In making ethical decisions, the health care practitioner must focus on two important considerations. First, as an individual, you can make ethical decisions only for yourself. To attempt to force your ethical choices on someone else is to attempt to force your value system on that individual. Would you want that done to you? Probably not. When you feel the need to intervene in the ethical decision-making process of someone else, it is permissible to act as an advocate by providing your viewpoint and all the available supporting information. However, if you do this, you have an ethical obligation to listen to the other person's viewpoint and allow him or her to make a decision without further interference.

One exception to the rule of only making ethical decisions for oneself is the parent–minor child relationship. Until children can distinguish between right and wrong, parents have an obligation to make ethical decisions for them. This obligation is based on the traditional principle of paternalism. The second consideration is that many ethical decisions are made quickly without much of an opportunity to analyze and rethink all the options. Therefore, the health care practitioner must be well prepared with a basic framework by which he or she can quickly make decisions that will seem wise and sensible long after the crucial moment.

## Ethical Autonomy

In health care, a debate often centers on who should have ethical autonomy. The debate is moot since the only person who can have ethical autonomy is the individual faced with the ethical dilemma. Also, the debate misses the point of what ethical decision making is all about. Ethical decision making is not about deciding what is best for someone else, it is about resolving ethical dilemmas for oneself. Nevertheless, the debate continues.

The ethical autonomy debate often manifests itself in statements such as "Why should respiratory care practitioners concern themselves with ethical dilemmas when the physician will make the final decision?" There is some truth in the statement; the physician *will* make the final decision about many patient care issues. However, the physician's decision is a legal rather than an ethical right. Each health care professional group has a legal scope of practice. Within their legal scope of practice, the practitioner is obligated to perform certain tasks and to make certain decisions about patients.

As leaders of the health care team, physicians have the broadest scope of practice, which puts them in the role of making many of the most visible and sometimes most critical patient care decisions. To the extent that these decisions attend to ethical dilemmas, studying ethics will assist other professionals, like respiratory care practitioners, in understanding the ethical resolution.

## PARTICIPATING IN ETHICAL DECISION MAKING

### Ethics Committees

In an attempt to deal with the rapidly increasing number of ethical dilemmas as well as to avoid litigation, over the past decade many hospitals and long-term care facilities have formed ethics committees. Fittingly, it was one of the most controversial ethical cases that caused the birth of ethics committees in hospitals and related institutions: the 1976 New Jersey Supreme Court ruling on Karen Ann Quinlan.[3]

Considerable activity took place following the New Jersey decision; however, it was not until 1991 that the Joint Commission of Accreditation of Health Care Organizations mandated the establishment of some mechanism to consider ethical issues in patient care and to educate health care professionals and patients in these issues. These mechanisms, or committees, are also sometimes called ethics review boards. Their purpose is to provide consultation to the health care team.[4] Consultations are usually provided in those cases where consensus cannot be reached by health care team members. These committees bring an abundance of resources to the resolution of ethical conflict and the ethical decision-making process. Committees have procedures under which their services can be requested. This information should be well known to all members of the health care team. There is no typical list of cases that might be considered by ethics committees since these committees generally become involved only on the request of someone close to a case that presents a difficult ethical dilemma. By default, however, this means that ethics committees often deal with cases involving life support, allocation of resources, and the futility of care.

Ethics committees are generally empowered only to issue recommendations. These recommendations may be accepted or rejected by the health professionals directly involved in delivering patient care. The following quote from the American Medical Association Judicial Council governs the recommendations of most ethics committees. "The recommendations of the Ethics Committee should be offered precisely as recommendations imposing no obligation for acceptance on the part of the institution, its governing board, medical staff, attending physicians or other persons."[5]

In addition to assisting the health care team in resolving major ethical dilemmas, the ethics committee typically serves the general function of establishing a general ethical code of behavior. It may also serve a review function as an ethical quality control measure. For example, one or two patient charts may be reviewed monthly or quarterly to determine in retrospect if appropriate ethical guidelines had been followed. The general duties of an ethics committee are:

- Provide staff development educational activities about potential ethical dilemmas
- Develop a set of policies, procedures, or guidelines for recognizing and resolving ethical dilemmas
- Serve as a clearinghouse for information on ethical dilemmas and resolution
- Serve as a forum for discussion and debate on ethical dilemmas and resolution
- Provide options or recommendations in specific cases
- Serve as a source of support for those involved in ethical dilemmas

The makeup of ethics committees varies widely. Typically, a well-rounded committee will be made up of one or more representatives from the medical staff, administration, nursing, ancillary services, risk management, medical social work, and the clergy. A medical ethicist is also generally on the committee. This person may be someone from the above group with a special interest in ethics or an ethics professor from a nearby university. The role of the medical ethicist is to serve as a resource person for the committee. He or she must be well-versed in ethical principles and theories as well as trends in ethical decision making.

Additional committee members should include non-health care professionals. High-level executives or members of the institution's board of trustees generally should not serve as a committee members. It is extremely important that the membership be balanced in such a way that the committee does not become a rubber stamp for wishes of the institution or any other special-interest group. It is also important that committee members feel free to express their views without fear of repercussions of any sort. Training and development of committee members is an important component of the committee's existence. Outside trainers and consultants should regularly facilitate discussions of ethical principles, theories, and dilemmas.

Committee size is also important. An extremely large committee will be unmanageable, and yet the committee must be large enough to provide a broad range of perspectives when considering ethical dilemmas.[6] A good size for most institutions is around a dozen members. The average number of meetings per year is about seven.[7] The success of ethics committees is unclear at this point. Researchers are only now attempting to measure the success of these committees. A major difficulty is determining what criteria should be used as a measure of success.

## Decision Making as a Process

Medical ethics experienced a major transformation in the late 1960s and early 1970s.[8] This is evident in part in the movement away from approximately a dozen relatively rigid traditional ethical principles to a less definite list of five or six contemporary principles. The movement has been gradual and not related to any specific school of thought. Rather, it has been somewhat reflective of concurrent changes in society. To some extent, the transformation is still ongoing; however, the major shift of moving ethical decision making from a procedure to a process seems to be complete. Prior to the transformation, ethics was seen as a list of prescriptive statements focusing on what should and should not be done.

Physicians were seen as the sole ethical decision makers for medical ethics. Opinions of nonmedical personnel were disregarded on the premise that in order to make decisions about medical ethics, one had to be knowledgeable about medicine. With the formation of ethics committees, it has become clear that although technical and medical knowledge is important when making medical-related ethical decisions, broad-based knowledge from other areas is also extremely important. With limited imagination, it should now be abundantly clear that individuals from all walks of life may have something significant to contribute to the ethical decision-making process.

Although the stated objective of ethical decisions was to promote the well-being of the patient, the patient was not given an opportunity to influence the decision. In fact, deceiving and manipulating the patient was considered quite acceptable as long as it was "for the patient's benefit." Thus, overall, ethical decision making was nothing more than a procedure to be followed when certain situations arose.

Since the transformation, ethical decision making has become more of a process. Participants are not only interested in the final decision but also in the rationale for the final decision. The rationale is open to question to determine its validity in each situation. All members of the health care team participate in the ethical decision-making process. Additionally, nonmedical personnel are very involved in the process. In fact, one of the hallmarks of the process is the importance placed on the need for the process and outcome to be understandable to nonmedical personnel.

The patient is now a major participant in the process. Although the patient is not invited into the conference room, great effort is taken to include what the patient needs and wants as part of the outcome of the decision-making process. Patient self-determination is considered to be an important component in the process along with benefit to the patient.

## The Individual Decision-Making Process

Ethics committees do not relieve the individual from the responsibility of making ethical decisions. One of the major objectives of this book is to systematically provide for the reader the tools needed for individual ethical decision making. Chapter 3 describes how beliefs, values, and morals impact the view that individuals have of ethical principles. Chapter 5 details the most common currently used ethical theories. Chapter 6 describes the commonly accepted ethical principles along with an approximation of the weights typically assigned to them. At that point, the reader will theoretically have the tools necessary to make sound ethical decisions.

The missing ingredient is the reasoning process the decision maker applies to the ethical question. The following discussion is intended to raise the reader's awareness of this important ingredient. The philosophical concepts from which this discussion was taken are much broader than what is presented here. In the interest of brevity, only those points necessary to this discussion are described.

From a philosophical standpoint, a question or issue may be empirical or evaluative. Simply speaking, empirical evidence is something that appears to be factual based on observation. This should not be taken to mean that empirical evidence is necessarily true. In fact, empirical evidence may indeed be false. For example, a health care practitioner may conclude that a patient is dying. The conclusion, if based on objective evidence of laboratory data and other patient conditions that signal dying in other patients, would be an empirical statement. However, as we all know, there is nothing absolute about the signs of dying. In fact the statement that a patient is dying may also be evaluative if it is not based on objective data. Evaluative statements are those which are made based on at least some subjective input. One of the major tasks decisions makers have prior to applying the ethical theories and principles is to examine their reasoning processes. That is, they must be able to determine whether their statements are empirical or evaluative. As illustrated in the example above, this is not always an easy task. However, the following clues can assist you in the process.

1. Empirical statements tend to use terms like "is," "was," or "will be."
2. Empirical statements tend to use terms that are defined in absolute terms rather than relative terms. For example: "The patient has a respiratory rate of 60 breaths per minute" versus "The patient has a rapid respiratory rate." "Sixty breaths per minute" is an absolute measurement. "Rapid respiratory rate" is a relative measurement.
3. Evaluative statements tend to focus on the quality or relativeness of something.
4. Evaluative statements tend to use terms like "good," "bad," "should," and "should not."[9]

Following are two lists of statements that respiratory care practitioners are likely to encounter in their work. The first list has been labeled and an explanation given as to why it is an empirical or evaluative statement. The second list is for the reader to use for practice.

### List 1: Empirical and Evaluative Statements—Examples

1. *The patient is experiencing tachycardia. (empirical)* "Tachycardia" is clearly defined in medical terms. It means a heart rate in excess of 100 beats per minute.
2. *The patient is in respiratory distress. (evaluative)* "Respiratory distress" is a widely used medical term, however, the meaning is not always specific. There are some objective measures of respiratory distress such as respiratory rate, blood gas results, and breathing patterns. However, there are no clear guidelines for combining this information and concluding that respiratory distress exists. The above statement can be changed from evaluative to empirical by deciding how the objective measurements will be used.
3. *The patient is suffering. (evaluative)* Suffering is obviously a subjective term. Its meaning is assigned by the user.
4. *The patient wants to die. (evaluative)* This statement draws a conclusion about the patient. Even if it appears to be supported by objective data such

as the patient's refusal to eat, it remains evaluative because the patient may have some other objective in mind. The only way the statement can be changed from evaluative to empirical is by a statement from the patient as in example 5 below.

5. *The patient has stated a desire to die. (empirical)* This statement illustrates both the simplicity and weakness of empirical statements. The statement may be clearly true; however, the message communicated may be totally false. It is not uncommon for people to make statements they do not mean.

**List 2: Empirical and Evaluative Statements—Practice**

*Directions:* (1) Determine whether each of the following statements is empirical or evaluative. (2) Explain your answer.

1. The patient has no quality of life.

2. This patient is experiencing acute respiratory failure.

3. This patient will never be weaned from the ventilator.

4. This patient should not be resuscitated.

5. This patient cannot sleep in a recumbent position.

## ✓ APPLIED EXERCISES

1. Develop three empirical and three evaluative statements. Explain why you classified each statement as you did.
2. Check the local hospitals in your community to see if they have ethics committees. If they do, what is the composition of the committees?

## STUDY QUESTIONS

1. What requirements must a decision maker meet to make sound ethical decisions?

2. Who has the responsibility for making ethical decisions for patients?

3. Why is there a decreasing emphasis on the issue of ethical autonomy?

4. What is the typical composition of an ethics committee? Why are nonmedical personnel included on medical ethics committees? Do you think nonmedical personnel should be included on ethics committees? Why or why not?

5. What are the major differences between how medical ethics was viewed prior to the transformation of the late 1960s and the early 1970s and after the transformation?

6. What is the difference between empirical and evaluative statements?

7. *Give an example of an empirical statement that may later be proved to be evaluative.*

8. *Should decisions made by ethics committees be binding? Why or why not?*

## REFERENCES

1. Beauchamp, TL, and Childress, JE: Principles of Biomedical Ethics. ed 2. Oxford University Press, New York, 1983.
2. Bankowski, Z: A code of ethics. World Health, January–February 1990.
3. Macklin, R, and Kupfer, RB: Hospital Ethics Committees: Manual for a Training Program. Albert Einstein College of Medicine, New York, 1988.
4. Manual for Ethics Committee Members. Froedtert Memorial Lutheran Hospital and John L. Doyne Hospital, Milwaukee, WI, 1994.
5. Judicial Council, American Medical Association: Guidelines for ethics committees in health care institutions. JAMA 253:2698–2699, 1985.
6. Glaser, J: Biomedical ethics: An overview. Paper presented at the Intensive Ethics Seminar for Pharmacy Faculty, Omaha, NE, October 1989.
7. McCarrick, PM, and Adams, J: Ethics Committees in Hospitals (Scope Note 3). Georgetown University, Kennedy Institute of Ethics, Washington, DC, 1987.
8. Finn, J, and Marshall, EL: In Garell, D (Ed): Medical Ethics. Chelsea House, New York, 1990.
9. VanDeVeer, D, and Regan, T (Eds): Health Care Ethics. Temple University Press, Philadelphia, 1987, p 5.

## ADDITIONAL SUGGESTED READINGS

1. La Puma, J, and Schiedermayer, D: Ethics Consultation: A Practical Guide. Jones and Bartlett, Boston, 1994.
2. Fleetwood, J, and Unger, SS: Institutional ethics committees and the shield of immunity. Ann Int Med 1:263–267, 1994.
3. Blake, DC: The hospital ethics committee—Health care's moral conscience or white elephant? Hastings Center Report 22:6–11, 1992.

# CHAPTER 5

# *Ethical Principles*

**Ethical Principles: The Basis of Health Care Ethics**
**Differing Views of Ethical Principles: Traditional Versus Contemporary**
**Traditional and Contemporary Ethical Principles and Their Meanings**
Autonomy
Beneficence
Confidentiality
Fidelity
Justice
Nonmaleficence
Paternalism
Quality of life
Reparation
Sanctity of life
Utilitarianism
Veracity
**A Patient's Bill of Rights**

## ETHICAL PRINCIPLES: THE BASIS OF HEALTH CARE ETHICS

Various researchers in the area of ethics have developed a list of ethical principles.[1] Twelve of these principles, a combination of both traditional and contemporary principles, are discussed here. These principles are important in the application of the ethical theories discussed in the next chapter. Each of these principles carries different weights, or values, for the ethical decision maker and thus will be applied differently in specific situations.

## DIFFERING VIEWS OF ETHICAL PRINCIPLES: TRADITIONAL VERSUS CONTEMPORARY

Ethicists may not agree on the number nor the meaning of the ethical principles. Further, the principles now viewed as being important are not those which were valued in years past. For example, prior to the 1970s, a dominant principle in health care was paternalism: There was a pervasive view that the medical establishment, primarily physicians, knew what was best for patients. Yet, in contemporary books on medical ethics, paternalism is seldom mentioned.

The major reason that paternalism has all but disappeared from the list of contemporary ethical principles is not that it no longer exists or is no longer practiced but primarily that the 1970s and 1980s brought a greater emphasis on autonomy. Since some health care professionals view autonomy as the opposite of paternalism, the difficulty in emphasizing the two principles concurrently is apparent. Other health care providers argue that paternalism is a protection of autonomy because it prevents patients from making decisions that may result in harmful consequences.[2] In the 1990s, the principle of autonomy has remained at the forefront of ethical problems. However, autonomy is gradually being overshadowed by the principle of justice as the primary ethical priority.[3] Within this principle lie the two components that are at the root of greatest debate in health care today: universal access and allocation of resources.

## TRADITIONAL AND CONTEMPORARY ETHICAL PRINCIPLES AND THEIR MEANINGS

It is important for the student of health care ethics and ethical decision making to be knowledgeable about both traditional and contemporary ethical principles. Neither the existence of traditional principles nor their influence disappears simply because ethical priorities change. Therefore, the remainder of this chapter is devoted to a description of common ethical principles, both traditional and contemporary. The common ethical principles, traditional and contemporary, agreed on by most ethicists are listed in alphabetical order in Table 5–1.

Table 5–1. TRADITIONAL AND CONTEMPORARY ETHICAL PRINCIPLES*

| TRADITIONAL | CONTEMPORARY |
|---|---|
| Paternalism | Autonomy |
| Quality of life (Meaningful) | Beneficence |
| Reparation | Confidentiality |
| | Fidelity |
| | Justice |
| | Nonmaleficence |
| | Sanctity of life |
| | Utilitarianism |
| | Veracity |

*Agreement on these distinctions is not complete.

## Autonomy

The principle of *autonomy* deals with the ability to govern one's self. It is considered to be a universal truth that everyone who has the ability to express his or her desires has a right to autonomy. The major exceptions to this principle are children who are unable to communicate and those who are otherwise mentally incompetent. It is the principle of autonomy, in part, that gives a patient the right to refuse treatment and to leave the health care institution without medical consent. This principle comes into conflict with the legal system when the expression of one's autonomy interferes with the autonomy rights of someone else. Otherwise, our society, on a theoretical level, health care institutions included, has been very accepting of our autonomy rights in recent years. In actual practice, however, many institutions, including many health care facilities, are often quite paternalistic in their practices. The simplest example of autonomy is a patient making a decision about his or her own care even if it is not in keeping with recommendations from health care practitioners.

## Beneficence

The principle of *beneficence* means that we should always do good for those we serve, in our case—patients. Since in health care we cannot always be certain that our procedures and therapy will do good, we have extended to the meaning of beneficence the precept that we will at least do no harm—an application of the principle of nonmaleficence. The difficulty with the principle of beneficence stems from the concept of doing what is good. There is very often major disagreement between individuals about what is good. Very often we as health care professionals assume we know what is good for a patient although the patient may totally disagree. The line between beneficence and paternalism becomes very thin when health care professionals begin to think in this fashion.[4] If you are ever faced with a similar situation, you should remember the principle of autonomy. That is not to imply that you should not attempt to reason with patients when you sincerely believe you have information that will benefit the patient. Note that the emphasis is on *benefiting the patient*, as opposed to knowing what's best for the patient. Any procedure done to a patient should be an example of beneficence.

## Confidentiality

The principle of *confidentiality* is generally an easy one to understand but sometimes quite difficult to apply. Very simply it means that information entrusted to us in the line of duty should not be revealed to others except when necessary for us to carry out our duty. In short, information should be made available only to those who "have a need to know." This principle carries considerable weight from a legal standpoint. It is especially important when dealing with the identity of patients and certain disease processes, for example, human immunodeficiency virus. The principle of confidentiality also carries great weight among health care practitioners. It is also probably the principle that is most often inadvertently violated. For example, any comment made about a patient in the hearing of anyone who does not have a need to know is a violation of that patient's right to confidentiality. Anyone walking quietly through almost any hospital in the country can observe a violation of this principle several times a day.

## Fidelity

The principle of *fidelity* deals with loyalty and may be defined as an obligation, or faithfulness, to duty. As a health care professional, employed by a health care institution, the worker has a responsibility not only to take care of patients but also to take care of patients to the best of his or her ability. For example, a worker may not wish to work with patients who have certain diseases, but the principle of fidelity would prohibit the worker from choosing to serve only certain patients. This principle is very important in legal considerations since it is often used as a benchmark in evaluating what an ordinary person might have done. Some modern-day practitioners may consider this principle to be old-fashioned; however, it is generally still given a significant amount of weight by most health care professionals.

## Justice

The principle of *justice* is also an easy one to define but is a difficult one to carry out. It states that everyone is entitled to equal care. The equality of care refers both to access to care and the level of care. Although most practitioners try to adhere to this principle, in reality all patients do not receive equal care, either in terms of access or in terms of level of care. Such factors as the type of insurance, age of the patient, social status of the patient, and so on routinely impact the equality of patient care. A major obstacle in applying the principle of justice equally is the lack of adequate funding for health care in general. As mentioned earlier, this principle is clearly at the forefront of our current health care reform efforts.

## Nonmaleficence

The principle of *nonmaleficence* is the opposite of the principle of beneficence. Specifically, it means to not inflict harm. As you have probably concluded, it is this principle that is at the base of most lawsuits. Most health care professionals strive not to cause harm to their patients, and generally when harm is caused it is not intentional. However, every medical procedure carries some risk. Thus it becomes the responsibility of the health care professional to evaluate whether the risk outweighs the benefit. Even with careful evaluation, some harm may occur, and the health care worker may incur liability. It is this principle that makes it extremely important that health care practitioners carefully evaluate the decisions they make as they deliver health care services.

*Ethical Principles* **55**

## ✓ APPLIED EXERCISE 5-1

Now that we have briefly discussed six of the twelve principles, a brief evaluation of your understanding is in order. This evaluation will give you the opportunity to explore some of the professional health journals. For each of the first six principles, which are listed again below, define the principle and then look for an example of each principle in a professional journal. Your instructor can make suggestions as to which journals you may use and where they may be found. Briefly summarize the examples below and discuss them with a fellow student or a working health care professional. You may also review the popular literature for examples.

### 1. Autonomy—Definition

_____
_____
_____

Example

_____
_____
_____
_____
_____

### 2. Beneficence—Definition

_____
_____
_____

Example

_____
_____
_____
_____

### 3. Confidentiality—Definition

_____
_____
_____

Example

## 4. Fidelity—Definition

Example

## 5. Justice—Definition

Example

## 6. Nonmaleficence—Definition

Example

_____

_____

_____

_____

You can check your examples in part by determining whether they fit the definitions. However, you should seek confirmation from an instructor or professional in your area of study. The discussions will assist in solidifying an understanding of the ethical principles. Remember, the purpose here is not that you simply rewrite the definitions but that you enhance your understanding by working with and discussing the definitions. For your benefit, the definitions are summarized below.

*Autonomy*—The quality or state of being self-governing

*Beneficence*—The act of doing or producing good

*Confidentiality*—The process of not sharing information with others unless they have a legitimate need to know

*Fidelity*—The obligation to duty

*Justice*—The act or process of providing equal treatment to all

*Nonmaleficence*—The act of preventing harm

The process of summarizing the definitions, finding examples, and discussing your understanding of the ethical principles is an extremely important part of developing ethical decision-making skills. Be sure to spend as much time as needed carrying out these tasks. When you are satisfied with your understanding of the first six principles, continue to study the last six principles.

## Paternalism

The principle of *paternalism* is one that your parents were bound by when you were a young child. Paternalism means to protect someone from his or her own judgments. The assumption is that the protector is more knowledgeable than the person being protected and thus will make the best decisions for all concerned. In health care the assumption is that as a skilled professional, you are more knowledgeable of disease and therapeutic processes than the patient. The actual application of this principle, however, is diminishing, clearly in theory and to some degree in practice. There has been a significant increase in the amount of self health care among patients who affirm their right to autonomy in deciding the direction of their health care. As autonomy increases, paternalism must decrease. As a future health care professional, you should also know that you are legally limited in your ability to insist that patients agree with your recommendations.

## Quality of Life

*Quality of life* is probably the most discussed of all the ethical principles. Although it is not often mentioned as one of the contemporary ethical principles, the current debate over the issue of assisted suicide indicates that this principle is alive and well. The difficulty with this principle lies in its definition. The principle implies that if there is no quality to life, then life is not worth living. The problem lies in attempting to define what is actually meant by "quality of life." Many individuals are alive but lack major bodily functions or survive only by means of life support equipment. Surrounding these individuals is often an ongoing debate about whether they have a meaningful quality of life. Very often the individual involved is not in a position to provide input, and thus it is often the family members and health care professionals who are left to debate the issue of quality.

As stated earlier, this principle receives considerable weight from a discussion standpoint but very little weight from an application standpoint due to the difficulty in arriving at a good working definition. When decisions about patient care, especially in regard to terminating life support, are made, they are usually made from a sanctity-of-life rather than a quality-of-life point of view.

## Reparation

*Reparation* is an easy principle to define. It means that there is an obligation to repair any harm caused to others either accidentally or on purpose. The problem in applying this principle in the health care setting is that very often it is impossible to repair the harm. For example, if a patient scheduled for an amputation of the right leg has the left amputated by mistake, it will be impossible to replace the left leg. Thus in such a case, the principle cannot be applied. It is usually with this principle in mind that courts award extremely large sums of money to victims of irreparable harm. Of course, the medical industry opposes this practice on the basis that there is some risk to every procedure and that liability should be limited when things go wrong. This principle should be weighted very heavily by health professionals although it is not often considered strongly until legal problems arise.

## Sanctity of Life

Of all the principles, *sanctity of life* probably weighs heavier on the minds of health care providers than any other. This principle means that life has value and must be preserved. It is this principle that creates the most conflict with the quality-of-life principle. It also creates some conflict with the autonomy principle. Sanctity of life is one of the most widely accepted values in our society. It affects many of the decisions we make and the actions we take. It also has a strong *legal* basis since it is clearly illegal, in most cases, to take the life of another person. From a quality-of-life standpoint, even if there is some agreement that a desirable quality of life is absent for a person, the sanctity of life makes it extremely difficult to permit any action that may result in shortening life. (This is true even in cases where the legal issue may not be the major problem.) Part of the problem is that sanctity of life comes into conflict with the autonomy principle, which in this case would say that only the individual involved really has the right to judge whether indeed there is quality of life.

The classic example of the application of this principle is the debate as to whether to preserve life at all cost.

## Utilitarianism

The eleventh principle, utilitarianism, is considered to be both an ethical principle[5] and an ethical theory.[6] *Utilitarianism* means that the greatest good should be done for the greatest number of people. As technology and the cost of health care continue to increase at an astronomical rate, this principle is becoming more and more important. Applied alone, this principle may actually prevent the development of new technology because it could be argued that money spent on research or on testing a new procedure or piece of equipment that would benefit only a small number of patients could be better spent taking care of a larger number of patients with existing technology. One example of this narrow-application technology is the artificial heart. Very few people have benefited from this extremely expensive procedure. However, researchers believe that eventually many will benefit. In the meantime, some patients may go without more conventional cardiac care because of the lack of funds to pay for this care.

Utilitarianism also conflicts with the sanctity-of-life principle. Because of our society's belief in the sanctity of life, we often expend large sums of money keeping individuals alive on life support equipment when it is quite clear that they will survive for only a limited period of time. Advocates of the utilitarianism principle would argue that this money could be used more effectively giving health care to someone who is likely to live longer. Of course, if this approach was always taken, new technology would never be developed. This principle is likely to remain a controversial one for some time to come.

## Veracity

The final principle is veracity. *Veracity* is honesty. It is one of the most widely held values in our society. There is a tendency, however, to distinguish between telling the truth in all cases and altering the truth in those cases in which the facts may be harmful. Sometimes in health care, patients are not told the complete truth about their diagnosis or prognosis. Family members will often request that their loved ones not be told or in some cases the physician may decide not to be totally truthful with the patient. Health care providers who are not primary care providers—for example, respiratory therapists or medical technologists—often avoid applying this principle by deferring the question to the patient's attending physician. This is acceptable because the patient's primary relationship is with the physician, and it is generally considered unethical for subordinate health care professionals to interfere with this relationship even if they know the true answer to the question. Licensing practice acts also very often prohibit subordinate health care professionals from making a diagnosis or issuing a prognosis; thus it is generally wise to avoid certain patients' questions.

Overall, the principle of veracity carries considerable weight in ethical decision making. In addition to the health care professional–patient relationship, it also ap-

**60** *Foundations and Issues*

plies to interaction among health care workers. It is even involved in cases where one professional may observe incompetent or unprofessional behavior on the part of another professional. Again, some licensure practice acts assign to each licensee the responsibility of being truthful and of reporting any inappropriate practice on the part of a fellow professional.

Now that we have discussed the last six ethical principles, it is time for another applied exercise. This applied exercise is identical to the assignment for the first six principles. You should define each of the principles in the space below and give an example of each. Remember to look for examples in the appropriate professional journals and discuss them with working professionals. Once you have located examples, be sure to discuss them with your instructor, fellow students, or professionals in your area of study. Good luck.

## ✓ APPLIED EXERCISE 5–2

### 7. Paternalism—Definition

_____
_____
_____

Example

_____
_____
_____
_____
_____

### 8. Quality of Life—Definition

_____
_____

Example

_____
_____
_____
_____
_____

## 9. Reparation—Definition

Example

## 10. Sanctity of Life—Definition

Example

## 11. Utilitarianism—Definition

Example

**12. Veracity—Definition**

_____
_____

Example

_____
_____
_____
_____

    Again, check your examples by looking to see if they fit the correct definitions. However, you should confirm them with your instructor or with a working professional. The definitions are summarized below for your review.

*Paternalism*—To act as a parent or to protect someone from his or her own bad judgment

*Quality of life*—The value or goodness of one's life

*Reparation*—The obligation to repair any harm whether accidentally or purposely inflicted

*Sanctity of life*—The belief that life has a high value and is to be preserved

*Utilitarianism*—The obligation to do the greatest good for the greatest number of people

*Veracity*—The value of being honest and telling the truth

    To this point, this chapter has introduced you to both traditional and contemporary ethical principles. Many of these principles will be discussed further in greater detail in following chapters.

## A PATIENT'S BILL OF RIGHTS

Another major guiding principle that defines for health care practitioners the manner in which they should interact with patients is the "Patient's Bill of Rights" (Box 5–1). This document was adopted by the American Hospital Association in 1972. As you will see, it incorporates many of the concepts expressed in the ethical principles.

## ✓ APPLIED EXERCISES

If you have made it this far in the chapter, you have completed the applied exercises. Congratulations!

### Box 5–1. A PATIENT'S BILL OF RIGHTS*

Effective health care requires collaboration between patients, and physicians, and other health care professionals. Open and honest communication, respect for personal and professional values, and sensitivity to differences are integral to optimal patient care. As the setting for the provision of health services hospitals must provide a foundation for understanding and respecting the rights and responsibilities of patients, their families, physicians, and other caregivers. Hospitals must ensure a health care ethic that respects the role of patients in decision making about treatment choices and other aspects of their care. Hospitals must be sensitive to cultural, racial, linguistic, regligious, age, gender, and other differences as well as the needs of persons with disabilities

The American Hospital Association presents a *Patient's Bill of Rights* with the expectation that it will contribute to more effective patient care and be supported by the hospital on behalf of the institution, its medical staff, employees, and patients. The American Hospital Association encourages health care institutions to tailor this bill of rights to their patient community by translating and/or simplifying the language of this bill of rights as may be necessary to ensure that patients and their families understand their rights and responsibilities. The following rights are included:

1. The patient has the right to considerate and respectful care.
2. The patient has the right to obtain from his physician and other direct caregivers relevant, current, and understandable information concerning diagnosis, treatment, and prognosis. Except in emergencies when the patient lacks decision-making capacity and the need for treament is urgent, the patient is entitled to the opportunity to discuss and request information related to the specific procedures and/or treatments, the risks involved, the possible length of recuperation, and the medically reasonable alternatives and their accompanying risks and benefits.

   Patients have the right to know the identity of physicians, nurses, and others involved in their care, as well as when those involved are students, residents, or other trainees. The patient also has the right to know the immediate and long-term financial implications of treatment choices, insofar as they are known.
3. The patient has the right to make decisions about the plan of care prior to and during the course of treatment and to refuse a recommended treatment or plan of care to the extent permitted by law and hospital policy and to be informed of the medical consequences of this action. In case of such refusal, the patient is entitled to other appropriate care and services that the hospital provides or transfer to another hospital. The hospital should notify patients of any policy that might affect patient choice within the institution.

4. The patient has the right to have an advance directive (such as a living will, health care proxy, or durable power of attorney for health care) concerning treatment or designating a surrogate decision maker with the expectation that the hospital will honor the intent of that directive to the extent permitted by law and hospital policy. Heath care institutions must advise patients of their rights under state law and hospital policy to make informed medical choices, ask if the patient has an advance directive, and include that information in patient records. The patient has the right to timely information about hospital policy that may limit its ability to implement fully a legally valid advance directive.
5. The patient has the right to every consideration of privacy. Case discussion, consultation, examination, and treatment should be conducted so as to protect each patient's privacy.
6. The patient has the right to expect that all communications and records pertaining to his or her care will be treated as confidential by the hospital, except in cases such as suspected abuse and public health hazards when reporting is permitted or required by law. The patient has the right to expect that the hospital will emphasize the confidentiality of this information when it releases it to any other parties entitled to review information in these records.
7. The patient has the right to review the records pertaining to his/her medical care and to have the information explained or interpreted as necessary, except when restricted by law.
8. The patient has the right to expect that within its capacity and policies, a hospital will make reasonable response to the request of a patient for appropriate and medically indicated care and services. The hospital must provide evaluation, service, and/or referral as indicated by the urgency of the case. When medically appropriate, and legally permissible, or when a patient has so requested a patient may be transferred to another facility. The institution to which the patient is to be transferred must first have accepted the patient for transfer. The patient must also have the benefit of complete information and explanation concerning the need for, risks, benefits, and alternatives to such a transfer.
9. The patient has the right to ask and be informed of the existence of business relationships among the hospital, educational institutions, other health care providers, or payers that may influence the patient's treatment and care.
10. The patient has the right to consent to or decline to participate in proposed research studies or human experimentation affecting care and treatment or requiring direct patient involvement, and to have those studies fully explained prior to consent. A patient who declines to participate in research or experimentation is entitled to the most effective care that the hospital can otherwise provide.

11. The patient has the right to expect reasonable continuity of care when appropriate and to be informed by physicians and other caregivers of available and realistic patient care options when hospital care is no longer appropriate.
12. The patient has the right to be informed of hospital policies and practices that relate to patient care, treatment, and responsibilities. The patient has the right to be informed of available resources for resolving disputes, grievances, and conflicts, such as ethics committees, patient representatives, or other mechanisms available in the institution. The patient has the right to be informed of the hospital's charges for services and available payment methods.

The collaborative nature of health care requires that patients, or their families/surrogates, participate in their care. The effectiveness of care and patient satisfaction with the course of treatment depend, in part, on the patient fulfilling certain responsibilities. Patients are responsible for providing information about past illnesses, hospitalizations, medications, and other matters related to health status. To participate effectively in decision making, patients must be encouraged to take responsibility for requesting additional information or clarification about their health status or treatment when they do not fully understand information and instructions. Patients are also responsible for ensuring that the health care institution has a copy of their written advance directive if they have one. Patients are responsible for informing their physicians and other caregivers if they anticipate problems in following prescribed treatment.

Patients should also be awsare of the hospital's obligation to be resonably efficient and equitable in providing care to other patients and the community. The hospital's rules and regulations are designed to help the hospital meet this obligation. Patients and their families are responsible for making reasonable accommodations to the needs of the hospital, other patients, medical staff, and hospital employees. Patients are responsible for providing necessary information for insurance claims and for working with the hospital to make payment arrangements, when necessary. A person's health depends on much more than health care services. Patients are responsible for recognizing the impact of their lifestyle on their personal health.

Hospitals have many functions to perform, including the enhancement of health status, health promotion, and the prevention and treatment of injury and disease; the immediate and ongoing care and rehabilitation of patients; the education of health professionals, patients, and the community; and research. All these activities must be conducted with an overriding concern for the values and dignity of patients.

*These rights can be exercised on the patient's behalf by a designated surrogate or proxy decision maker if the patient lacks decisionmaking capacity, is legally incompetent, or is a minor.*

*Reprinted with permission of the American Hospital Association, 1992.

**66** *Foundations and Issues*

## STUDY QUESTIONS

*1. Briefly respond to the following statement: There is a well-defined set of ethical principles that is widely agreed to be appropriate for use in all ethical decision making.*

*2. Which ethical principle was dominant in health care prior to the 1970s? What happened to diminish its dominance?*

*3. Which ethical principle appears to be exerting the primary dominance in the 1990s? Why?*

*4. The original Patient's Bill of Rights was written in 1972. It was revised in 1992. Do you think that the current transformation that health care is undergoing will require many of the principles to change in less than 20 years from 1992 in order to be current and applicable?*

## REFERENCES

1. Beauchamp, TL, and Childress, JE: Principles of Biomedical Ethics, ed 2. Oxford University Press, New York, 1983.
2. Fromer, MJ: Ethical Issues in Health Care. Mosby, St Louis, MO, 1981, p 316.
3. Veatch, RM: Cross Cultural Perspectives in Medical Ethics: Readings. Jones and Barlett, Boston, 1989, p 289.
4. Fromer, MJ: Ethical Issues in Health Care. Mosby, St Louis, MO, 1981, p 317.
5. Veatch, RM: Cross Cultural Perspectives in Medical Ethics: Readings. Jones and Barlett, Boston, 1989, p 197.
6. VanDeVeer, D, and Regan, T (Eds): Health Care Ethics. Temple University Press, Philadelphia, 1987, p 29.

## SUGGESTED ADDITIONAL READINGS

1. Jonsen, AR, Siegler, M, and Winslade, WJ: Clinical Ethics, ed 3. McGraw-Hill, Health Professions Division, New York, 1992.
2. Shortell, SM, and Kaluzny, AD: Health Care Management—Organization Design and Behavior, ed 3. Delmar, Albany, NY, 1994.

# CHAPTER 6

# *Ethical Theories and Methods*

The Deontological Theory
The Utilitarian Theory
The Analysis Method

Volumes can be written on ethical theories, subtheories, and nuances thereof. In doing so, ethicists and philosophers continue to define and add to our knowledge of ethics, behavior, and ethical decision making. The objective of this chapter is not to add to this vast field of knowledge, but rather to provide the reader with a basic understanding of the theories and methods used in making ethical decisions in health care. It is that objective that gives the author the liberty to include the "analysis method" on an equal level with theories in a chapter that focuses on ethical theories. The analysis method is nothing more than a decision-making process that combines the best of the two dominant ethical theories with practical problem-solving methods. In reality, it is probably the most practical ethical decision-making technique. Let's start this chapter by attempting to advance your understanding of the composition and functions of theories.

A theory can be defined as a set of rules or principles designed for the study or practice of an art or a discipline. Theories are not absolute in that they do not always work as expected. Theories are not static. What may appear to be a sound theory at one point in time may be modified as new information is discovered. There may be competing theories designed to explain the same situation.

Ethical theories are probably more vulnerable than many of the more traditional scientific theories. As illustrated in Box 3–1, ethical thinking is based on such imprecise and ever-changing concepts as personal belief systems, attitudinal orientation, personal value systems, and moral philosophies. Ethical theories are also more difficult to test since the best outcome may not be known for an extremely long time following an event. Even then, the best outcome can be debatable.

Ethical theories should be viewed as a guide for solving ethical dilemmas. Since there is more than one ethical theory, the problem solver must select the theory that appears to best fit the ethical dilemma at hand. In reality, in most cases the problem solver will actually select the theory with which he or she is most comfortable.

Ethical theories are bodies of ethical principles grouped in such a way that they create a system. These theories are useful in establishing a framework for solving ethical problems. They are based on ethical principles as well as on the value system of the person utilizing the theory. Ethical principles were discussed in Chapter 5. Two major theories, deontological and utilitarian, have been formulated for dealing with ethical dilemmas.[1]

## THE DEONTOLOGICAL THEORY

The word "deontological" is derived from the Greek *deontos,* meaning "duty." As discussed earlier, this theory is closely associated with the philosopher Immanuel Kant. Kant lived in Germany between 1724 and 1804. It is thought that Kant believed in the concept of absolute morality. Because of the focus on absolute morality, Kant's thinking does not involve itself with consequences; therefore, the theory is sometimes referred to as the nonconsequentialist theory. The deontological theory is also sometimes referred to as a formalist theory.[2]

The core of the *deontological theory* is its emphasis on the rightness or wrongness of a situation.[3] Therefore, in using this theory, the user must accept the concept that some things are inherently right or inherently wrong. This type of thinking draws heavily on the moral philosophy component of the foundation concepts of personal ethics discussed in Chapter 3. In a nutshell, morals define what we consider to be right and by implication what we consider to be wrong.

The deontological theory also relies heavily on the ethical principles, which are used to affirm the rightness or wrongness of a situation. Thus, when an ethical problem is discovered and the deontological theory is to be used, the following steps must be taken:

1. Identify the ethical principle or principles that support the concept of rightness or wrongness in the situation. This is not always easy to do; however, the validity of the final solution will depend on success with this step.
2. List all the alternative actions that possibly could be taken to solve the ethical dilemma. Compare each alternative action to each ethical principle identified in step 1. If only one alternative action and one ethical principle could apply and if each is consistent with the other, the problem is solved by taking the alternative action. If there is more than one ethical principle or alternative action, go to step 3.

3. If more than one ethical principle could apply, use the principle that carries the greatest weight—if that can be determined. Since ethical principles carry different weights for different people, the principle that carries the greatest weight for the person involved will be used.
4. Continue the process of comparing alternative actions to ethical principles until the alternative that is consistent with the highest ethical principle is identified.

If the highest ethical principle cannot be singled out or if an alternative that is consistent with it cannot be identified, the deontological method fails. A worksheet for this method might appear as follows:

**Ethical Dilemma**

_____
_____
_____
_____

Alternatives
(1) _____
(2) _____
(3) _____
(4) _____

Ethical Principle(s) Supporting Each Alternative
(1) _____
(2) _____
(3) _____
(4) _____

**Alternative(s) Consistent With Highest Ethical Principle**

_____
_____
_____

**Solution**

_____
_____

The following example illustrates how this method works.

> A respiratory care practitioner discovers that a patient is dumping part of the medication that is being placed in his medication nebulizer. When confronted, the pa-

tient acknowledges what he is doing explaining that he doesn't like the taste of the medication. He then asks the practitioner not to mention his actions to anyone else. The medication is essential in correcting a highly resistant respiratory tract infection.

In selecting the deontological theory to resolve this problem, the practitioner would have to accept the belief that there are some inherent rights or wrongs. He or she would also have to believe that this situation is one in which rightness or wrongness applies. Having accepted the deontological theory as being the proper tool for resolving this dilemma, the next step is to begin developing alternatives to the action desired by the patient.

The alternatives are: (1) honor the patient's request and forget the issue or (2) tell the patient's physician and write this information in the patient's chart. Choice 1 is supported by the autonomy principle. Choice 2 is supported by the fidelity and possibly the beneficence principle. The veracity principle also applies and probably carries the greatest weight of all the applicable principles; therefore, the solution would be to inform the patient's physician and chart the information. The veracity principle more than supports your action. The fidelity and beneficence principles add additional support. This dilemma was a relatively easy one. Many practitioners might question the need to work through a theoretical process to resolve this relatively minor ethical dilemma. To these practitioners, there is no real dilemma and no need to develop alternatives. To them, the answer was clear; there was no need for debate. In reality, even these practitioners actually used an ethical theory for making the decision that they simply knew to be right: They simply did not consciously work through the process. Let's look at a more difficult ethical dilemma.

A respiratory care practitioner enters a patient's room to perform an arterial blood gas puncture. The patient has a tracheostomy tube in place and is attempting to pour water into it. As the respiratory care practitioner enters, the patient abruptly stops his efforts and pleads with the practitioner to say nothing.

The alternatives are: (1) honor the patient's wish and say nothing, (2) report this incident so that the patient can be observed more closely, or (3) not report the patient but take on the personal responsibility of watching the patient more closely. Choice 1 is supported by the autonomy principle. Choice 2 is supported by the sanctity-of-life and the nonmaleficence principles. Choice 3 is supported by the paternalism principle.

The solution lies in the sanctity-of-life principle, which clearly carries the greatest weight; therefore, the practitioner should report the incident in order to have the patient observed more closely. Let's look at one more ethical dilemma.

While at the nurse's station checking a chart for some needed information, a respiratory care practitioner notices that the patient has a diagnosis of human immunodeficiency virus (HIV). Shortly thereafter she discovers that the person is a friend of a friend who apparently does not know about the HIV diagnosis. Her first temptation is to tell her friend.

The alternatives are as follows: (1) Tell the friend. As she contemplates this action, she is unable to find an ethical principle to support her intended action. (2) The other choice is to not tell her friend. This choice is supported by the principle of confidentiality. The solution lies in the principle of confidentiality. The practitioner should not tell her friend. It is extremely important to adhere to the principle of confidentiality.

As presented here, the decision-making process is extremely simple using the deontological theory. Of course, the dilemmas presented here are also extremely simple. In fact, the dilemmas are so simple that most practitioners would be able to make a decision easily without specifically considering ethical theories or principles. On the other hand, when dilemmas are presented that are not so clearly right or wrong, the deontological theory becomes potentially more difficult to use.

## THE UTILITARIAN THEORY

The second major ethical theory to be discussed is sometimes referred to as one of the traditional ethical principles. The utilitarian theory is actually one of the teleological theories. The teleological theories differ from the deontological theory in that the consequence of actions is considered. As a result, the teleological theories are sometimes referred to as the consequentialist theories. The utilitarian theory is the most common of the teleological theories. It is closely associated with nineteenth-century British philosophers John Stuart Mill and Jeremy Bentham.[4]

The core of the *utilitarian theory* is the emphasis on accomplishing the greatest good or utility. A great deal of attention is focused on the value of happiness, or the greatest good. In fact, some advocates of this theory maintain that the end, if it is desirable and good, justifies the means even if they are less than desirable. The theory differs significantly from the deontological theory in that is does not acknowledge the rightness or wrongness of a situation. In fact, using this theory might make it acceptable to engage in what might otherwise might be viewed as a wrong act provided the act produced the highest happiness value relatively to the other alternatives. This possibility produces what is considered by many to be a major flaw in this theory.[5]

In applying this theory the following steps are followed after an ethical dilemma has been identified.

1. List alternatives that appear to be better than the current action.
2. Predict the consequences of each alternative and assign a happiness value to each alternative.
3. Select the alternative that has the highest happiness value and use it as the ethically correct choice.

It should be noted that there was no attempt to match the alternatives to the ethical principles to make any comparison among the ethical principles. This method fails if acceptable alternatives cannot be identified, if consequences cannot be predicted accurately, or if happiness values cannot be estimated accurately.

A worksheet for this method of analysis might appear as follows:

**Ethical Dilemma**

_____
_____
_____
_____

Alternatives
(1) _____
(2) _____
(3) _____
(4) _____

**Consequences of Each Alternative**

_____
_____
_____
_____

**Happiness Value for Each Alternative**

_____
_____
_____

**Alternative With the Highest Happiness Value and the Ethically Correct Choice**

_____
_____
_____

Following is an example of this method in use:

> During a prenatal examination, Mrs. Jones's physician discovers an open genital herpes lesion. He advises her that if an open lesion is present at delivery, the virus may be transmitted to the child. He tells her that he plans to note this on her chart. Mrs. Jones pleads with the physician not to put the information in the chart explaining that, as the wife of the mayor of a small town, the information would almost certainly become public and would embarrass the family.

**List of Alternatives**
1. The physician could ignore Mrs. Jones's request and place the information on the chart.

2. The physician could leave the information out of the chart but make a note in a place accessible only to him since he would be the one delivering the baby.

**Consequences of Each Alternative**
1. This alternative would cause unhappiness to the Jones family and possible damage to Mr. Jones's political career.
2. This alternative would harm no one and would bring great happiness to the Joneses.

**Happiness Value for Each Alternative**
1. Extremely low
2. High

The alternative with the highest happiness value and the ethically correct choice is 2: Do not place the information on Mrs. Jones's medical chart.

Again, resolution of this ethical dilemma, as presented, using the utilitarianism theory was quite simple. However, whether the solution was the correct one is open to question. There also may be a legal problem for the physician in failing to chart this information. Legally or ethically, what if the physician were out of town and someone else had to deliver the baby and did not know to take the appropriate precautions? What about other medical personnel that may be exposed? Does the solution still appear to be so simple? There will be ample opportunity to discuss these questions later!

## THE ANALYSIS METHOD

In addition to the two ethical theories, there is also a major problem-solving model that can be used for ethical dilemmas as well as for other problems. This model is referred to by some as a *step-by-step analysis*. It does not utilize the ethical principles directly; however, since the problem solver's value system will come into use as possible solutions are evaluated, the ethical principles are used indirectly. The method attempts to lead the problem solver to a logical and workable solution. In the early stages of the analysis, the method gives the problem solver several options to quit the process if the problem cannot pass an initial evaluation.

The steps in the analysis method are:
1. Recognition and identification of the problem
   a. What is the context of the data source(s)? If the context is inappropriate, exit from the process.
   b. Is the data source reliable? Accurate? Logical? If not, exit from the process.
   c. Is the perceived problem really the problem? If not, exit from the process.
   d. Whose problem is it? If it is not the problem solver's problem, exit from the process.

2. Clarification of the problem
   a. Conceptualization—In what context is the problem to be analyzed? What approach(es) (ethical theories) can be used to analyze the problem? What is the best approach to use? What ethical principles are involved with this problem?
   b. Prioritization—What is the priority of the problem from an organizational viewpoint? What is the priority of the problem from the problem solver's viewpoint?
   c. Solution—What is the best solution from an organizational viewpoint? What is the best solution from the problem solver's viewpoint? Which viewpoint has the greatest priority? Apply the solution with the greatest priority.

It is easy to see that the analysis method is nothing more than a problem-solving model designed to ensure that the problem is treated systematically. There are both positive and negative benefits to using this method. From a positive standpoint, the user may be able to avoid possible emotions or biases that may be evoked by involvement of the ethical theories prior to clarification of the problem. From a negative standpoint, since ethical principles are not mentioned early in the problem-solving process, the user may fail to use them or may use only selected principles. The result may be an attempt to solve an ethical problem for a patient (acting paternalistic) as opposed to solving the problem for the user. To some degree, using the deontological or utilitarian theories as problem-solving methods forces the user to consider the appropriate ethical principles in all phases of the problem-solving process. In reality, however, the analysis method is likely the most popular approach to resolving ethical dilemmas.

Now, let's use the analysis method to consider the two ethical dilemmas presented as examples for the deontological and utilitarian methods. In the first example, a respiratory care practitioner discovers a patient dumping medication. That, of course, is not the ethical dilemma. Medication dumping by the patient is simply a patient care problem. The dilemma occurs when the patient asks the respiratory care practitioner to conspire with him and not mention it to anyone. Obviously, if the respiratory care practitioner could have convinced the patient to take the medication, the ethical dilemma would have been avoided.

The first step in the analysis method is recognition and identification of the problem. If the therapist simply sees the problem as directing the patient to take the medication, the therapist may become paternalistic (without giving any thought to ethics) at this point. On the other hand, if the therapist sees the problem as convincing the patient to take the medication, she or he will have entered the realm of ethical problem solving, that is, she or he will have recognized the existence of an ethical dilemma. At least two ethical principles would immediately come to bear: fidelity and autonomy.

The patient in this case, however, rapidly moved the context forward to one of fidelity and veracity for the therapist by requesting that the information be kept secret.

At this point, all the questions in step 1 can be answered and summarized:
   a. What is the context of the data source? The patient is providing the data directly. There is no hearsay or speculation.

b. Is the data source reliable? Accurate? Logical? The therapist observed the patient not taking his medication and was further requested by the patient to withhold this information. This is the most reliable and accurate type of information one can have. The events are logical.
c. Is the perceived problem really the problem? Yes, the therapist has identified the correct problem. Patient compliance is at the root of the problem; however, the most immediate problem is the ability of the practitioner to maintain faithfulness (fidelity) to his duties and to be truthful (veracity) in the context of the patient's right to autonomy.
d. Whose problem is it? While the ultimate problem of patient compliance may not be that of the practitioner, the immediate dilemma of fidelity and veracity is the practitioner's.

In step 2 of this process, the problem solver will actually begin to seek a solution to the dilemma.

a. Conceputalization: In what context is the problem to be analyzed?
The problem has to be analyzed in the context of the practitioner's duty to deliver care to this patient.
What approach(es) can be used to analyze the problem?
The approaches available to the therapist in this case include gathering additional information, involving others, or proceeding with the information already available. Other than attempting to determine why he is refusing the medication and seeking recommendations for a different medication, the practitioner seems to have all the information needed. If the practitioner decides to involve someone else at this point, she or he will have violated the patient's autonomy in such a manner that might preclude further trust from the patient. Note: there is no intent to suggest here that the practitioner is so obligated to honor the patient's request that no one else can be involved. If this were the case, there would be no ethical dilemma; however, the problem of the patient's compliance would continue to exist. The practitioner would in essence be caught in an "ethical trap." The point is that whether to involve others is part of the ethical dilemma.
What is the best approach to use? The best approach in this case is to determine which ethical principles are involved and the relative weight that each principle will carry. What ethical principles are involved with this problem? The ethical principles that are clearly apparent here include the principle of autonomy on the part of the patient and veracity and fidelity on the part of the practitioner.
b. Prioritization: What is the priority of the problem from an organizational viewpoint? Extremely high. The patient is hospitalized for treatment. The practitioner, as an agent of the hospital, has the responsibility to deliver the treatment. What is the priority of the problem from the problem solver's viewpoint? Extremely high. This is not just a matter of the practitioner needing to "do the job." At issue here is the practitioner's faithfulness to duty and obligation to be truthful.

c. Solution: What is the best solution from an organizational viewpoint? Failure of the patient to comply with the treatment would constitute a failure of the organizational mission. On the other hand, an outright rejection of the patient's right to autonomy would also be a failure of the organizational mission. In short, the organizational mission needs to be preserved in both cases. What is the best solution from the problem solver's viewpoint? In this case, the organizational viewpoint and the problem solver's viewpoint are identical. This will not always be the case. In fact, in a large number of cases, it is the conflict between the organizational and problem solver's viewpoint that creates the ethical dilemma. Which viewpoint has the greatest priority?

Since the viewpoints are the same, there is no need to answer this question. Apply the solution with the greatest priority.

It's clear in this case that the patient needs to comply with the treatment plan. The right to autonomy is extremely important; however, this is not the arena in which it should be asserted. The practitioner must be faithful and truthful. The patient can choose to refuse treatment; however, it must be done openly and recorded in his records.

It may appear on first impression that the analysis problem-solving method is more complex than the deontological or utilitarian methods. In fact, it is more involved in terms of the number of steps or questions that must be answered; however, it is the method most commonly used. It also has a major advantage over either of the two other methods individually: It allows the problem solver to select components of the deontological or utilitarian methods as appropriate. As a result, the problem solver is more likely to arrive at an ethical conclusion that is acceptable to everyone involved.

##  APPLIED EXERCISES

The ability to use any ethical problem-solving method depends on the ability to clearly understand the process through application. These decision-making processes are used routinely even in cases where decision makers may be unaware of how they arrived at their conclusion. Because they are not aware of a systematic process, decision makers may experience unnecessary distress both during and after making the decision. The likelihood of arriving at an acceptable solution is also decreased when the process is not systematic.

For this applied exercise, the learner should review issues of local newspapers for the most recent two or three weeks. (Back copies can be found in the library.) The objective is to find at least three articles, preferably medically related, in which an ethical decision was made. As best as can be determined from the news account, identify the decision-making process used. See if you can relate the decision-making process to those discussed in this chapter. Write down your findings and discuss with classmates or other practitioners.

## STUDY QUESTIONS

1. Briefly explain why ethical theories may be more vulnerable to criticism than more traditional scientific theories.

2. Which ethical theory considers the consequences of an action resulting from decisions made using the specified theory?

3. Which of the ethical theories discussed in the chapter is more closely associated with the concept of absolute morality?

4. Which of the ethical theories discussed in the chapter is more closely associated with accomplishing the greatest good or utility?

5. On a practical basis, in your opinion, which theory or method is most likely to be used to solve ethical problems? Why or why not?

## REFERENCES

1. Beauchamp, TL, and Childress, JE: Principles of Biomedical Ethics, ed 2. Oxford University Press, New York, 1983.
2. VanDeVeer, D, and Regan, T (Eds): Health Care Ethics. Temple University Press, Philadelphia, 1987, p 34.
3. Purtilo, R: Ethical Dimensions in the Health Professions. ed 2. Saunders, Philadelphia, 1993, p 10.
4. VanDeVeer, D, and Regan, T (Eds): Health Care Ethics. Temple University Press, Philadelphia, 1987, p 29.
5. Ibid, p 32.

## ADDITIONAL SUGGESTED READINGS

1. Lammers, S, and Verhey, A (Eds): Introduction. In On Moral Medicine: Theological Perspectives on Medical Ethics. Eerdmans, Grand Rapids, MI, 1987.
2. Ackerman, TF, and Strong, C: A Casebook of Medical Ethics. Oxford University Press, New York, 1989.

PART

TWO

*Applications and Practices*

CHAPTER 7

# *Applied Ethical Decision Making*

**Case Studies**
Case Study 3: The High-Risk Infant
Case Study 4: The Secret Smoker
Case Study 5: The Tardy Physician
**Discussion**

In this chapter the respiratory care practitioner will be introduced to applied ethical problem solving using the principles and theories discussed in the previous two chapters. The practitioner may note in these case studies that one may face an ethical dilemma even though one is not in position to make a final decision about the outcome of the identified problem. To that end, the practitioner should remember that one can only make ethical decisions for oneself. There is a mistaken belief in many cases that making the right ethical decision always leads to the one best solution for everyone involved.

## CASE STUDIES

### Case Study 3: The High-Risk Infant

Sam S. is a registered respiratory therapist with a Bachelor of Science degree. He is employed in a large training hospital where a wide range of patients are cared for. He has a special interest in neonatal care and is certified by the National Board for Respiratory Care (NBRC) as a neonatal therapist. For the past year Sam has served as the lead therapist in the neonatal unit.

The ethical dilemma in this case centers on a 12-day-old infant who was born after 26 weeks of gestation. The infant is suffering from idiopathic respiratory distress syndrome, which is not responding to surfactant replacement therapy. Clinical evaluation also shows that the infant is suffering from a cardiac malfunction of unknown severity. The infant has received continuous respiratory care since birth. The infant's unmarried mother does not appear to understand the seriousness of the situation and has not been asked to participate in the decision-making process about the future of her child. The health care providers have slowly arrived at the conclusion that the prognosis is somewhat hopeless. The neonatologist, however, is willing to continue treatment for the time being in spite of the prognosis since there is still some slight hope that the infant can survive. There are several major concerns about each possible course of action.

A clinical conference is held in an effort to decide what should be done in this case. Participants are the chief neonatologist, the medical social worker, the clinical nurse specialist for neonatology, and Sam S., representing respiratory care. The hospital does not have an active ethics committee. Each participant in the conference expresses various concerns and viewpoints. The neonatologist shares her concern that further treatment may be futile, expensive, and excessively time-consuming, with an extremely poor prognosis. She emphasizes that if the infant survives, extensive care is likely to be needed during the infant's first few months at home—possibly longer. The medical social worker expresses serious concern about the well-being of the child if it survives and is discharged to the mother. He has investigated the family situation of the mother and is very discouraged. The mother is unemployed, except for sporadic temporary work that does not provide a steady source of income. The nurse specialist expresses displeasure at continuing the seemingly futile treatments. She points out that this infant's diagnosis is similar to several other infants who died after months of expensive and time-consuming treatment. She feels that the infant should gradually be weaned from all life support equipment, allowing nature to take its course. Sam S. is asked to share his concerns and opinions. Sam partially shares the concern expressed by the nurse; however, he also feels a strong obligation to continue the treatment.

A discussion ensues among the participants. Issues from the ethical principle of justice dominate the conversation. It quickly becomes obvious that the issues of allocation of resources and the seeming futility of continuing care will play major roles in deciding the outcome of this situation.

## The Learner's Solution

*To the Learner:* Without purposely referring to the ethical principles or theories, briefly, in the space below, describe how you would resolve this dilemma.

_____
_____
_____
_____
_____
_____
_____
_____
_____
_____
_____
_____
_____
_____

## The Deontological Solution

The first step in the deontological solution is to identify the ethical principle or principles that support the concept of rightness of wrongness of the situation. (Note: Only contemporary ethical principles will be used in the decision-making process; however, the traditional principles may be used in the discussion of the process and solution.)

1. The principles that appear to be appropriate here include fidelity and justice. The second step involves listing the alternative actions that might be taken to resolve the ethical dilemma and then comparing those actions with the ethical principles identified in the first step.
2. Possible alternative actions:
   a. Continue maximum treatment for the infant. This action would be supported by the principle of fidelity and the component of the principle of justice that requires equal treatment for all.
   b. Decrease treatment to a minimum. This action might be supported by the component of the principle of justice that says resources should be allocated fairly. One could argue, however, that this component may actually support leaving the infant on the life support equipment.

For this case, the deontological problem-solving process would end at this point. However, two strong ethical principles support continuing maximum treatment for the infant. There is only weak support from a component of the justice principle for decreasing treatment to a minimum. Therefore, the decision has to be to continue maximum treatment. Remember, the deontological method does not consider consequences, it only looks at the "rightness" of the situation as it exists at the moment.

## *The Utilitarian Solution*

The first step in the utilitarian solution is to list the alternatives that appear to be better than the current action. The assumption is that if the current action were the best solution, no dilemma would exist. This step also reveals one of the weaknesses of the utilitarian method—lack of agreement as to what the alternatives to the current method are.

1. Alternatives to current action:
   a. Decrease treatment to a minimum level.
   b. Educate the mother on the expected prognosis and involve her in the decision-making process.
   c. Provide maximum care for those ailments which are responding positively to care, and decrease care to the nonresponding ailments.

The second step in the utilitarian method requires an even more difficult task than the first step. In the first step, the problem solver must attempt to predict the consequences of each alternative and assign a happiness value based on the desirability of the consequences.

2. Consequences and happiness value of each alternative:
   a. If the treatment is decreased to a minimum, the likely consequence is that the infant will die. The happiness value here may be difficult to see. If there is a happiness value for this alternative, it is based on preventing a prolongation of futile treatment. This decision is likely to carry the highest happiness value for the nurse.
   b. If the mother is brought into the decision-making process, the likely consequence is that whatever decision is ultimately made will have her support. The decision made under these circumstances will likely have the highest happiness value for the mother.
   c. If maximum care is continued, there will be minimum happiness for anyone. Although the neonatalogist has expressed her willingness to continue maximum treatment, she has also expressed her concern that it is probably futile.

At this point, the best ethical decision appears to be to bring the mother into the decision-making process for two reasons. First, not to bring her into the process at this point would mean that the health care workers are proceeding to make ethical decisions for this patient (the infant) without any input from the party that is most affected. Remember, ethical decisions can be made only for oneself. The second reasons to involve the mother is to preserve her right to autonomy and justice. Given the appropriate information, the mother is likely to make a decision that will bring a high happiness value to all concerned. The ultimate outcome for the infant is not likely to change by bringing the mother into the decision-making process.

## *The Analysis Solution*

Although the solution from the analysis method should be very obvious at this point, selected steps will be considered briefly for illustrative purposes.
1. *Recognition and identification of the problem.* All items in step 1 have been dealt with clearly. There is indeed an ethical dilemma based on valid data, and the problem does belong in part to the health care team. It also belongs in part to the mother. One advantage of this method is that the mother would likely have been brought into the process at this point.
2. *Clarification of the problem.* The problem is being analyzed in the context of the patient's needs, the prognosis, and the health care facility and team's ability to provide care for this patient and other patients. The best approach to use is to gather all the information possible and be sure that all affected parties are involved. The ethical principles that must be considered are fidelity on the part of the health care team, autonomy on the part of the patient (the mother in this case), and justice on the part of all concerned.

    The priority of the problem from an organizational as well as the problem solver's viewpoint is high. The major concern for the organization is the efficient allocation of resources. In addition to allocation of resources, the problem solver must also be concerned with the three ethical principles identified above. Therefore, while the best solution from the organization's viewpoint would simply be to provide minimal care or to discontinue care altogether, this "best solution" is clearly outweighed by the problem solver's concerns. The best solution then continues to be one in which the mother is brought into the decision-making process preserving the problem solver's obligation to address the three identified ethical principles.

It should be noted that the analysis method allows the problem solver to use both the deontological and utilitarian methods as desired in solving dilemma. Therefore, it is clearly a superior method of resolving ethical dilemmas. The analysis method consists of nothing more than the basic steps for solving problems modified to deal specifically with ethical dilemmas. For the remainder of this book, this approach should be used in developing solutions to ethical problems. In some cases, minor modifications may need to be made to fit the specific ethical situation. As we work through the remaining chapters, the emphasis will be on developing additional information to improve ethical decision making and simultaneously to hone the skills for making these decisions. Since there is not necessarily a "correct" answer for any ethical dilemma—for example, the deontological and utilitarian answers may even differ significantly—readers will always be given a chance to develop their own solutions to the ethical dilemma. The author, in some cases, will then offer a solution as a guide to the way the problem might be approached. Thus, the emphasis is not on the one "correct" answer but, instead, on developing problem-solving skills.

## Case Study 4: The Secret Smoker

Staci W. is a rehabilitation and home care therapist. She works with patients in the rehabilitation clinic and performs follow-up with them at home. One of the specific classes Staci conducts at the rehabilitation clinic is smoking cessation. In one of her smoking cessation classes, Staci has a patient named Mr. Benjamin. He is in the class on the recommendation of his primary care physician. During the class, Mr. Benjamin is somewhat resistant to the idea of quitting smoking. He states several times to other patients that he is taking the class only to make his physician happy. He further relates that his physician has told him that he would not prescribe home oxygen therapy for him unless he quit smoking. Mr. Benjamin, who frequently complains of shortness of breath, wants badly to have oxygen at home. By the end of the class he indicates that he has quit smoking and thanks Staci for her help.

Three months later while filling in for another therapist, Staci visits Mr. Benjamin at his home. She finds Mr. Benjamin sitting on his front patio, with the oxygen temporarily turned off, smoking a cigarette. Staci expresses surprise. Mr. Benjamin shrugs his shoulders, states that he will never quit smoking, and demands that Staci not tell his physician.

*The Learner's Solution*

*To the Learner:* Without purposely referring to the ethical principles or theories, briefly, in the space below, describe how you would resolve this dilemma.

*The Analysis Solution*

1. *Recognition and identification of the problem.* The problem is this case is very clear, although not simple. Mr. Benjamin is not complying with his

treatment objectives, something which he has a right to do under the principle of autonomy. The dilemma is that he is asking Staci to conspire with him in his deceit, thus creating an ethical dilemma for Staci. The context is appropriate (Staci is dealing with the dilemma as part of the professional-client relationship). The data source is reliable and accurate (Staci observed Mr. Benjamin smoking, and he confirmed that he smokes and does not plan to quit). This is a real problem for several reasons: (1) Mr. Benjamin, who has oxygen at home, is creating a fire hazard by smoking. (2) Mr. Benjamin is negating the positive effects of the therapy by continuing to smoke. (3) Mr. Benjamin is not true to his primary care giver and is asking another care giver to conspire with him in the deceit.

Other problems may be involved that the reader can identify. If so, write them in the space below:

___

___

___

The ethical dilemma here belongs to Staci. (Mr. Benjamin also has an ethical dilemma; however, that is a separate issue from Staci's dilemma.) She must decide whether to keep Mr. Benjamin's confidence, giving him autonomy, or to reveal the information she has discovered to Mr. Benjamin's physician which is her professional duty.

2. *Clarification of the problem.* This problem must be analyzed in the context of Staci's relationship with her client and with the physician. It should be noted that Staci is, in essence, an agent of the physician in this case since the primary relationship here is between Mr. Benjamin and the primary care physician. This relationship defines the approach Staci must use in solving this problem. She has no choice but to approach the problem from the standpoint of a professional care provider and the associated responsibilities.

The ethical principles involved here include fidelity and autonomy. Other ethical principles may be involved. If the reader can identify any, write them in the space below:

___

___

___

___

The organization in this case is the medical community, specifically, the health care team and resources involved in providing care. Obviously, the priority of the problem from the organizational viewpoint is high. There is little point in providing care to Mr. Benjamin if he refuses to comply with the guidelines of that care. Furthermore, the issue of safety is prominent in this case.

From the organization's standpoint, Mr. Benjamin needs to be in compliance with his treatment objectives, one of which is that he will not smoke. Although there may not be an ethical principle that supports the organization's view, no other solution can possibly be considered.

Staci, the problem solver in this case, must wrestle with the competing principles of autonomy for the patient and fidelity for herself. One way in which she can approach this conflict is to invoke the principle of beneficence. This would lead her to the following conclusion: To allow autonomy for the patient would not only conflict with her need to be faithful to her duty, it would also cause harm to the patient. Therefore, her solution becomes clear. She cannot support the patient's demand for autonomy without carrying out her need to be faithful to her duty and attempting to benefit the patient. Staci reports the smoking to the attending physician. It should be noted that the patient is not being totally denied his right to autonomy. Mr. Benjamin can certainly continue to smoke; however, he cannot expect the health care provider to condone it either directly or indirectly.

## Case Study 5: The Tardy Physician

> June P. is a special procedures therapist in a medium-size for-profit hospital. Her duties include performing pulmonary function and pulmonary and cardiac stress tests. She enjoys her work tremendously since she gets to spend time and talk with her patients. Her dilemma stems from the behavior of one of the physicians with whom she performs cardiac stress tests. He is never on time for his scheduled patients. To add to her frustration, June is aware of the reason for this lateness—he is having an affair with another hospital employee. The real dilemma for June is that this physician always directs her to tell the patient that he is late because he has been held up by an emergency.

### *The Learner's Solution*

*To the Learner*: Without purposely referring to the ethical principles or theories, briefly, in the space below, describe how you would resolve this dilemma.

_____
_____
_____
_____
_____
_____
_____
_____

## The Analysis Solution

1. *Recognition and identification of the problem.* This is a complex ethical dilemma for June. It involves both her interaction with her patients and with the physician. The context and source of the data are clear since June is experiencing the problem directly as she works on a daily basis. The dilemma is causing June personal distress; therefore, it is clearly her problem.
2. *Clarification of the problem.* June has two relationships to consider as she conceptualizes this problem. In regard to the physician, she has an obligation to be an effective health care team member. In regard to the patient, she has an obligation to exercise the principle of veracity. There is also an issue of confidentiality in June's relationship with the physician. To put it bluntly, the affair that the physician is allegedly having is actually none of June's business and should not enter into the problem-solving analysis. Acknowledging the reason that the physician is late is actually not part of the ethical dilemma, and this simplifies the problem and allows June to view her relationship with the physician as a team member strictly on a professional level.

Although the priority of solving the dilemma from an organizational viewpoint should be high, in reality, the organization is unaware of the problem. If June follows the instructions given to her by the physician, the organization is never likely to become aware of the problem. The priority from the problem solver's viewpoint is high. The problem is creating frustration for June, causing her to be untruthful to her patients, and interfering with her ability to complete her job in a timely and efficient manner. June needs to move ahead and solve the problem.

The best solution from the problem solver's viewpoint is to not be untruthful to the patient. It should be noted that this does not mean that June should now tell the patient that the physician is late because he is having an affair. She definitely should not tell the patient this. The patient need only be told that June cannot say why the physician is late. She should also tell the physician what she will tell the patient. She will now have effectively removed herself from the "middle" position making the lateness issue one between the physician and the patient.

## DISCUSSION

It's likely that some of the solutions offered for the preceding dilemmas may not have been what was expected by the reader. In considering this, the reader should note two things. First, there is seldom full agreement on what is the best absolute solution to an ethical dilemma. However, the systematic ethical problem-solving process will lead to an acceptable solution when it is applied correctly. Second, very often when ethical dilemmas are approached, the problem solver may be attempting to resolve an issue which cannot be resolved or which is at least beyond his or her realm of power or influence. For example, in Case Study 4, getting the patient to quit smoking is not the ethical dilemma; however, the health care provider may see the smoking as the dilemma that must be resolved. Cast Study 5 presents a similar dichotomy. Regardless of how the therapist feels about the affair the physician is having, the affair is not the dilemma. Therefore, correctly, the solution to the ethical dilemma does not involve consideration of the affair.

Practice with the analysis method will eventually allow the learner to automatically and rapidly work through the problem-solving process and arrive at an acceptable solution. This method has several merits. First, it ensures that the problem is clearly identified, that the data are reliable and accurate, and that the problem belongs to the person attempting to solve it. Second, it places the problem in the appropriate context and assists the problem solver in determining the best approach and the ethical principles to be used. Third, it clarifies the priority of the problem from an organizational and problem solver's viewpoint. Finally, it leads to the best solution from the organizational and problem solver's viewpoint.

## STUDY QUESTIONS

### Short Answer

1. *Briefly contrast the approaches to ethical problem solving presented in the deontological, the utilitarian, and the analysis methods.*

2. *After having had the opportunity to view each of the ethical problem-solving methods in use, which method do you prefer? Why?*

### True/False

1. *An ethical dilemma can only exist when an individual is in a position to completely resolve it.*
2. *The ethical principle of justice means that treatment should be related to the patient's ability to benefit from the treatment.*
3. *In Case Study 3, since there is a general conclusion among most of the health care providers involved that the prognosis is extremely poor, it is clear, beyond doubt, that additional care in this case is futile.*
4. *In Case Study 3, the mother's poor economic status negates her right to autonomy.*

5. *For health care providers, the ethical principle of fidelity means that confidences shared with patients should be keep confidential.*

## SUGGESTED READINGS

1. Gorovitz, S (Ed): Moral Problems in Medicine, ed 2. Prentice-Hall, Englewood Cliffs, NJ, 1988.
2. Daugherty, CJ: American Health Care: Realities, Rights, and Reforms. Oxford University Press, New York, 1988.
3. Bok, S: Lying: Moral Choice in Public and Private Life. Pantheon Books, New York, 1978.

# CHAPTER 8

# *Confidentiality*

**The Issue**
**Legal Considerations**
**Ethical Considerations**
**Case Studies**
Case Study 6
Case Study 7

## THE ISSUE

Confidentiality is discussed in a separate chapter because it is one of the most significant issues encountered by health care professionals. Historically, in health care, the principle of confidentiality was derived from the principle of fidelity. It was assumed that if the health care practitioner was faithful to his or her duty, then the information that exchanged between the patient and practitioner would not be disclosed to anyone without the patient's permission.[1] The importance of confidentiality in health care was recognized in the following passage from the Hippocratic oath: "Whatever, in connection with my professional practice, or not in connection with it, I see or hear, in the life of men, which ought not to be spoken abroad, I will not divulge, as reckoning that all such should be kept secret."[2] Confidentiality also has a prominent place in the American Hospital Association's Patient's Bill of Rights (see Chapter 5). Thus, the principle of confidentiality has a long history in health care.

Although the image of the lone health care practitioner working diligently with a patient has changed significantly, with few exceptions it is still generally accepted that the information in a patient's medical record is privileged and should not be revealed to anyone unless that person has an absolute need to know. Codes of confidentiality, however, are not absolute. Under certain circumstances it may be not only desirable but necessary to break the code of confidentiality. Since the consequences for breaking the code can be serious, the respiratory care practitioner must know when it is ethically and legally appropriate to disclose patient information. This chapter will assist the respiratory care practitioner in dealing with the many dilemmas associated with maintaining confidentiality.

What is confidential information? All information about a patient, regardless of how it is obtained, is considered to be confidential. When confidentiality issues arise, new health care practitioners often immediately think of information which might be controversial or which the average person might want to keep hidden from public knowledge. However, regardless of whether it might be controversial, if it is information obtained from the patient or about the patient in the course of treatment, in most cases it should be treated as confidential. It is just as unethical to disclose information about a patient who is being treated for bronchitis as it is to disclose information about a patient being treated for AIDS. Therefore, maintaining confidentiality means more than not disclosing information that might be considered sensitive, it also means maintaining all patient information within the bounds of the "need to know."

When may confidences be broken? Attempts to answer this question have occupied many authors and ethicists.[3] There is no single, easy answer to the question. Generally speaking, breaking confidentiality is considered acceptable when the purpose is to prevent a harmful outcome or to promote a positive outcome. The reader should note that prevention of harm carries a heavier weight than the promotion of good probably because it may be easier to determine when harm has been prevented. Furthermore, the prevention of a specific harm to a specific individual or individuals carries more weight than the prevention of a general harm to unspecified individuals. Since it is not easy to know when harm will be prevented or good promoted, the effort to predict the outcome of an action is usually the source of the ethical dilemma. The following guide may be helpful in determining when it might be appropriate to break confidentiality. The reasons are listed in descending order of appropriateness: The first reason carries considerable weight, the second carries moderate weight, the third carries limited weight, and the fourth carries very little weight. Using these guidelines does not excuse the user from making an appropriate ethical decision.

It may be appropriate to break confidence when the result is:
- The prevention of a specific harm to specific individuals
- The prevention of a specific harm to nonspecific individuals
- The promotion of a specific good to nonspecific individuals
- The promotion of a nonspecific good to nonspecific individuals

The prevention of a specific harm to specific individuals is the rationale used by public health agencies requiring the reporting of conditions such as tuberculosis, child abuse, and sexually transmitted diseases, including AIDS, under certain circumstances. The specific preventable harm is clear and the specific individuals are either a family member, sex partner, or other easily identifiable individuals who will be harmed by a lack of knowledge regarding the condition. The prevention of a specific harm to nonspecific individuals may also apply here since in many cases, the individual at risk for harm may not be easily identified in advance.

Another consideration related to confidentiality is the need to preserve a patient's dignity and to promote the healing process. In almost every health care encounter, patients are called upon to disclose very private information about themselves. For some patients, understandably, the process of sharing private information with strangers produces anxiety and distress. If the patient cannot feel comfortable that personal information will be safeguarded, then the discomfort will likely to turn into distrust. There is every reason to believe that patient's response to treatment will be negatively affected if the patient is suffering from anxiety, distress, and feelings of distrust.

Some of the major problems currently threatening confidentiality involve the handling of computerized, stored medical records and managed care. Both computerized records and managed care bring to the health care industry convenience, efficiency, and reduced cost. The computerized record is likely more accurate, more transferable, and even more easily reproducible than the handwritten version. All these attributes enhance the delivery of managed care. Unfortunately, these attributes also make the information more easily accessible to individuals without a need to know the contents of the record.

## LEGAL CONSIDERATIONS

Maintaining information on patients in a confidential manner is a legal responsibility.[4] Although all health care practitioners who access the medical record in the course of carrying out their duties have a responsibility to safeguard the confidentiality of the medical record, health information practitioners have a special interest in this area since they are responsible for maintaining the record after discharge of the patient. In a position paper in 1993, the American Health Information Management Association attempted to establish the difference between confidential and nonconfidential information in the medical record. According to this position paper, confidential information includes, although is not limited to, all clinical data as well as the patient's address upon discharge. Data considered nonconfidential includes the patient's name, verification of hospitalization or outpatient services, and the dates of the delivery of service.[5]

Respiratory care and other health care practitioners, however, should not interpret this position paper to mean that it is acceptable to routinely disclose nonconfidential information. The distinctions drawn in the position are purely technical ones for use by health information practitioners as they safeguard the contents of the medical record. All citizens, including patients in the health care system, have a right to privacy. Although confidentiality and privacy have different meanings, their applications are quite similar when applied to medical information. Thus the routine disclosure of information such as the patient's name or verification of services along with dates may quickly begin to erode the confidentiality of the medical record.

There are certain legal exceptions to the requirement to maintain all patient information in strict confidence. Fortunately for respiratory care practitioners, these exceptions are primarily the responsibility of other members of the health care team. However, these exceptions will be discussed briefly here in order to ensure a clear understanding for everyone concerned.

The most common legal exception to the need for patient information confidentiality is when there is a legal requirement, usually a Public Reporting Statute, designed to ensure the collection of vital statistics and the reporting of communicable diseases and cases of child abuse or neglect and injuries that may have been inflicted under criminal conditions. The reporting of vital statistics is required simply in order to maintain accurate public records. This routine reporting is usually done by the health information management department of the hospital and consists of information such as birth and death certificates. If there is anything unusual about a death, an official such as a medical examiner will become involved and additional information including autopsy results may be involved in the report.

Several laws and regulations affect the confidentiality of medical records: the Privacy Act of 1974, the Conditions of Participation for Hospitals in Medicare and Medicaid Programs, the Conditions of Participation for Long Term Care Facilities and the Uniform Health Care Information Act. These laws and regulations are quite complex in some cases. In general, they both require and prohibit the disclosure of information in specific situations. Most of these laws and regulations are federal in nature, although many states have adopted similar requirements. For the respiratory care practitioner, adherence to the basic operating principle that all information is confidential and should not be disclosed without a need to know will ensure compliance with these various laws and regulations. The employing facility will develop and administer policies and procedures for dealing with the above laws and regulations as appropriate.

## ✓ APPLIED EXERCISE 8–1

Contact the health information management department of a local hospital or check the appropriate state statutes in your library, and obtain additional information on the requirement to report vital statistics in your state. Record the information below.

_____
_____
_____
_____
_____

Many states require the reporting of diseases that may be communicable or contagious. Typically, all the common childhood diseases are included as part of the statute in most states. In reality, many of these childhood diseases are not reported by private medical facilities. However, if treatment is rendered in public medical facilities or if large populations are in danger of being infected—for example, day care centers or schools—the diseases will likely be reported. Certain sexually transmitted diseases may be included as part of this category, for example, gonorrhea and syphilis. Many states are currently struggling with the need and utility of reporting infection with the human immunodeficiency virus. Most states have some type of reporting requirement currently in place.

## ✓ APPLIED EXERCISE 8–2

Contact your local health department or check the appropriate state statutes in your library, and list below the diseases that must be reported as part of the communicable disease reporting requirement in your state.

_____
_____
_____
_____
_____

In recent years, most states have implemented a requirement to report suspected child abuse or neglect. The statute usually applies to those individuals, including health care workers and teachers, who are in a position to notice abuse or neglect. With the current prevalence of child abuse in our society, this responsibility should not be taken lightly. It is also important not to overreact in these cases; therefore, it is extremely important for respiratory care practitioners to understand the reporting requirements in their states and the manner in which these requirements may affect them.

## ✓ APPLIED EXERCISE 8–3

Research the child abuse reporting statutes in your state. Summarize them in the space below.

_____
_____
_____
_____
_____

The final category usually required under the Public Reporting Statutes involves injuries that may have been inflicted under suspicious or criminal circumstances. Health care professionals primarily affected by this reporting requirement are pre-hospital care personnel (EMTs and paramedics) and hospital emergency room staff. There are additional conditions under which the requirement to maintain patient information in a confidential manner may be expected; however, they are beyond the scope of this book.

## ETHICAL CONSIDERATIONS

Respiratory care practitioners should keep in mind that even when patient information may become a part of the public record due to a legal requirement, they are not relieved of the responsibility to keep the information confidential from an ethical standpoint. Failure to do so will interfere with the professional relationship between the practitioner and the patient. An ineffective professional relationship might impede patient care. The longer or more intense the relationship the practitioner has with the patient, the more critical this concern becomes. For example, if the patient is in a home care setting or in a rehabilitation program, a major impetus to the patient's compliance with treatment is the trust and confidence shared by the health care provider and the patient.

From an ethical standpoint, the strict requirement of confidentiality on the part of the health care practitioner is related largely to the patient's right to privacy. Some ethicists see the right to privacy as an extension of the ethical principle of autonomy.[6] In this sense, it should be easy to understand a patient's right to control the disclosure of personal information. There is no reason to assume that patients give up this right when they submit themselves to a health care practitioner for treatment. In fact, as mentioned earlier in this chapter, the ethical principle of fidelity places on the health care practitioner the ethical responsibility of protecting patient care information.

## CASE STUDIES

### Case Study 6

Jody K., RRT, is shocked when she enters Room 1126. There is the odor of smoke—marijuana smoke. As she approaches the patient's bedside, a quick debate ensues in her mind. What should she say to the patient? Challenge him? Say nothing? Report the patient? She decides to ask the patient about the smell of smoke, not about marijuana. After all, she isn't totally sure what marijuana smoke smells like, and maybe she was mistaken about the odor.

Did Jody do the right thing? Using any or all of the ethical decision-making models, provide as much support as possible for Jody's decision.

If possible, devise an alternate solution to this dilemma. Record your support of Jody's decision and your own conclusion below.

## Case Study 7

Ashleigh W., a special procedures respiratory therapist, routinely checks the computer for information about her next cardiac stress test patient. To her surprise, there are no data for this patient in the computer. She rechecks the handwritten requisition and then calls the intensive care unit who had forwarded the request to the cardiopulmonary department. She is informed by the nurse that the patient is indeed there but that this is a "no publicity" case. It immediately dawns on Ashleigh why this is so as she again reads the patient's name on the requisition. The patient is a local candidate for political office who has been "unavailable for comment" for the past 24 hours. The election is this very day, and the patient has been hospitalized and is being tested for cardiac problems. The real problem for Ashleigh, however, is that the patient's opponent in the political race is the father of her very best friend. Ashleigh realizes that she has a piece of hot political information.

What should Ashleigh do with the information? Support your answer using either or all of the ethical decision-making models. Record your conclusions below.

## STUDY QUESTIONS

*1. What patient information should be considered confidential?*

*2. Is confidentiality a legal or an ethical responsibility?*

*3. From an ethical standpoint, why is confidentiality important?*

*4. What is the relationship between the ethical principles of autonomy and confidentiality?*

*5. What is the relationship between privacy and the ethical principle of confidentiality?*

## REFERENCES

1. Veatch, RM: Cross Cultural Perspectives in Medical Ethics: Readings. Jones and Bartlett, Boston, 1989, p 83.
2. Hippocrates. The Oath. In Hippocrates: Vol I (trans. by W. H. S. Jones, The Loeb Classic Library). Harvard University Press, Cambridge, MA, pp 299–301 (quote p 301), 1923.
3. Jonsen, AR, Siegler, M, and Winslade, WJ: Clinical Ethics. Macmillan, New York, 1982, p 154.
4. American Medical Association. Principles of Medical Ethics. AMA, Chicago, 1981.
5. American Health Information Management Association. Maintenance, Disclosure, and Redisclosure of Health Information. AMA, Chicago, 1993.
6. Annas, G, et al: The Rights of Doctors, Nurses and Allied Health Professionals. Ballinger, Cambridge, MA, 1981, p 172.

# CHAPTER 9

# Human Experimentation and the Use of New Technology

The Issue
Legal Considerations
Ethical Considerations
Case Study
Case Study 8

## THE ISSUE

Human experimentation is essential for the development of new procedures and technology to care for sick patients. Although animal research, simulation computer models, and other methods can be used extensively to project the impact of a new procedure, drug, or technology on patient care, the actual outcome cannot be determined until human subjects are used. There is nothing inherently improper in using human subjects in experimentation as long as certain conditions and requirements are met. From an ethical standpoint, the principles of beneficence, nonmaleficence, and justice must be carefully considered whenever the subject of human experimentation is addressed. The application of these principles in human experimentation will be discussed further in this chapter in the section on ethical considerations.

There are many examples of unethical human experimentation. One well-known example is the experimentation performed in the German concentration camps, which is representative of unregulated and uncontrolled human experimentation. Unfortunately, as horrible as these experiments were, they were not isolated instances. Recent reports have revealed that in the United States a major human experiment was undertaken without the consent and knowledge of the subjects involved. Specifically, in the early 1930s a study designed to observe the effects of untreated syphilis was carried out on uninformed African-American citizens in Macon County, Alabama, home of the Tuskegee Institute Hospital. Originally designed to last only 6 months, the study continued for 40 years. It ended only when the public press began to publish reports on the fate of some of the unwitting subjects and raise ethical questions. According to an ad hoc committee formed during the seventies by the Department of Health, Education, and Welfare, there were three key considerations: the issue of informed consent, the justification for conducting the study, and the question as to whether treatment should have been provided for the subjects. The committee also considered whether the study should be terminated.

The committee issued a report in 1973, which was widely considered to be flawed and which concluded that the major ethical error was the failure to provide treatment to the subjects. This ethical error was dismissed in part by pointing out that in 1932, there was no effective treatment for syphilis, although many physicians were using arsenic and bismuth to treat syphilitic patients. The committee apparently concluded that the subjects had been given informed consent for the study since they accepted token incentives such as hot meals and $50 for burial expenses.[1]

Although most incidents of human experimentation do not have a direct relationship to the delivery of respiratory care, it is essential that the respiratory care practitioner develop a clear understanding of the issues associated with human experimentation in order to avoid potential problems. When looking at cases of human experimentation, two terms must clearly be understood: common practice and experimental care. When procedures, treatments, or drugs are approved and applied on a regular basis by a wide range of qualified practitioners, they fall into the category of common practice. Experimental care, on the other hand, refers to those procedures, treatments, or drugs whose effectiveness has not been totally proved, that is, official approval usually has not been given. In the early days of respiratory therapy, respiratory care practitioners were often involved in procedures that had not been documented as being therapeutically sound. In that sense, respiratory care practitioners have been major participants in human experimentation. It should be noted that whenever a new piece of equipment, new procedure, or new bronchoactive drug is applied or administered in way that is different from its originally intended use, experimentation is taking place. Common areas in which respiratory care practitioners may find themselves involved on an experimental basis include:

1. Equipment modifications not approved by the manufacturer
2. Adaptation of equipment for new uses when the adaptation is not based on controlled research
3. Administration of medication via a mode different from that recommended by the manufacturer, for example, aerosolization of medication designed for injection
4. Administration of medication at a different frequency from that recommended by the manufacturer

> **Box 9–1. THE NUREMBERG CODE**
>
> *Principle One:* Voluntary consent of the human subject is absolutely essential. The person should have the legal capacity to give consent, and there should be exercise of free will with no element of force, fraud, or coercion. All the elements of informed consent must be present, and the duty for ascertaining the quality of consent rests with he individual who directs or conducts the experiment; it cannot be delegated.
>
> *Principle Two:* The experiment must be designed to yield fruitful results for the good of society that are not procurable by other means and that are not random or unnecessary in nature.
>
> *Principle Three:* The experiment should be based on the results of animal experimentation and on a knowledge of the natural course of the disease or problem. Anticipated results should justify performing the experiment.
>
> *Principle Four:* The experiment should be conducted so as to avoid all unnecessary physical and mental harm.
>
> *Principle Five:* No experiment should be conducted in which there is reason to believe that death or disabling injury will occur, except perhaps those in which the experimenting physicians also serve as subjects.
>
> *Principle Six:* The degree of risk to be taken should never exceed the humanitarian importance of the problem to be solved.
>
> *Principle Seven:* Precautions should be taken to protect subjects from even a remote possibility of injury or death.
>
> *Principle Eight:* The experiment should be conducted only by scientifically qualified persons who demonstrate the highest degree of skill and care throughout all stages of the experiment.
>
> *Principle Nine:* During the course of the experiment the subject must always be at liberty to discontinue participation if he has reached a point beyond which continuation will be physically or mentally harmful.
>
> *Principle Ten:* The scientist in charge must be prepared to terminate the experiment at any stage if he has probable cause to believe that continuation will result in injury, disability, or death of a subject.

It is not always easy to clearly identify what is experimental and what is innovative. The first comprehensive and probably most authoritative legal document that establishes legal guidelines for human experimentation is the Nuremberg Code (Box 9–1). This code resulted from the trial of 23 Nazi physicians following World War II. These trials focused on atrocities committed by the Nazis. Several charges were alleged in this war crimes trial, all of which dealt with human experimentation without informed consent. Although the physicians were charged with "crimes against humanity," they contended that they were performing medical experiments. Many of those charged with war crimes were convicted and sentenced to long prison terms or in some cases death.

The Code, consisting of 10 principles, provides guidelines for legal, ethical, and moral behavior in human experimentation.[2] Of the principles set forth in the Nuremberg Code, Principle 1, requiring that patients subjected to experimentation must give informed consent, is probably the most important.[3,4]

Informed consent carries weight as both a legal and an ethical doctrine and is a common concept in the practice of health care. It simply means that patients must always be informed as to the intent, the expected outcome, and the risk involved with any procedure or therapy. It can only be given by a patient who is legally competent, who has the power of choice, and who is able to comprehend the procedure to which they are consenting. The courts have been adamant in upholding the patient's right to informed consent. It should be noted that there is no test to ensure comprehension, at least in therapeutic settings. Thus the only absolute requirement in informed consent is one of disclosure. In an attempt to enhance the likelihood of comprehension, there is generally a requirement that the patient not be under the influence of drugs and that the disclosure is given in language that the patient is likely to understand.

## LEGAL CONSIDERATIONS

As mentioned in the discussion of the Nuremberg experiments, one of the most important legal considerations is informed consent. Experimentation, however, presents a unique challenge to the concept of informed concept. By its very definition, the risk involved in an experimental procedure is unknown. Furthermore, the expected outcome is purely theoretical. Only the intent can be stated with reasonable certainty. Many lawsuits have resulted from cases where there is a dispute over the extent to which the patient was correctly informed regarding the nature of the procedure. In an attempt to clarify what constitutes informed consent in human experimentation cases, the United States Department of Health, Education and Welfare has devised a set of guidelines that list the elements that must be present:

1. Fair explanation of the procedure to be followed, including identification of experimental methods
2. Description of attendant discomforts and risks
3. Description of the benefits to the subject that are expected
4. Disclosure of appropriate alternative procedures that might be advantageous to the subject
5. The offer to answer any inquiries concerning the procedure
6. Instruction that the subject is free to withdraw consent and discontinue participation in the project at any time.

As simple as these elements appear to be, they are far from being so. For example, in the first element, a "fair explanation" assumes that the experimenter and the patient will have a similar understanding of the procedure once the explanation is completed, but that is often not the case. It is impossible for the experimenter to explain clearly to a patient all of the nuances of the procedure of which he or she may be aware.

It is also very likely that there will be vocabulary and comprehension gaps between the two. Elements two and three present similar difficulties as element one.

Since the procedure is experimental in nature, descriptions of attendant discomforts, risks, and benefits can be nothing more than calculated predictions. The experimenter views these predictions from a broad base of knowledge, but the patient probably views them from a very different perspective.

## ETHICAL CONSIDERATIONS

Three key ethical principles are associated with human experimentation and informed consent: autonomy, beneficence, and nonmaleficence. The principle of autonomy is exercised by the patient, whereas the principles of beneficence and nonmaleficence become the responsibility of the health care provider. The general meaning of each of these principles is provided in Chapter 6.

The principle of autonomy, as related to human experimentation, ensures that a patient has a right to be in complete control of the type of treatment to which he or she is subjected. This principle maintains that, above all, the patient has the right to self-determination. Inherent in the patient's ability to intelligently exercise this right is the assumption that the patient will be informed of the purpose and side effects of a proposed treatment as well as the alternatives. In the case of the Tuskegee experiments, in order for the patients to have exercised autonomy, it would have been necessary for them to know that the course of treatment planned for them would likely result in a serious progression of their disease and possibly death. It would also have been necessary to inform them that there was an alternative treatment.

The second opportunity to avoid this kind of ill-fated experimentation lies with the health care provider. If the principle of beneficence and nonmaleficence had been observed by Tuskegee health care providers, they would have had to conclude the following:

- The experiment should be of direct benefit to the subjects upon whom it is being performed.
- Minimally, if benefit could not be absolutely ensured, the next obligation would be to ensure that the experiment would not bring harm.

It is clear that in the case of the Tuskegee experiments, the experimenters did not seriously consider either the principle of beneficence or nonmaleficence. In fact, their stated purpose was to study the long-term effects of the disease when left untreated. It is clear that this purpose violates both principles. Unfortunately, this type of behavior may continue to occur unless there is concentrated vigilance on the part of all health care practitioners. Respiratory care practitioners must do their part to guard against this type of behavior.

## APPLIED EXERCISE 9–1

Search as many editions of a major newspaper as necessary until you are able to locate five or six articles dealing with new or innovative medical procedures. Consider such procedures as gene therapy and laser surgery for the treatment of emphysema. Analyze the articles and prepare a discussion on the way researchers dealt with the ethical dilemmas that may have been created by their research.

## CASE STUDY

### Case Study 8

Jennifer R. is a special procedures therapist in a 250-bed hospital. Her duties consist primarily of performing cardiac and pulmonary stress testing and pulmonary function testing (PFT). In a continuous effort to upgrade equipment, the hospital decides to purchase a new PFT machine. The PFT company salesperson and technical representative comes to the hospital to install the equipment. After a half day of in-service training for Jennifer, she is left to operate the equipment alone. The next day she performs her first PFT on a patient. The results do not appear to be consistent with the patient's general condition based on Jennifer's experience, so Jennifer repeats the test. The second test results are essentially the same. Jennifer reports the results.

A few days later, the patient's physician calls and questions the results. Jennifer tells the physician that she too was concerned and had repeated the test. Although not completely satisfied, the physician accepts the results as reported. Jennifer, however, is still concerned and decides to call the PFT company's technical representative. After describing how she had conducted the test, the technical representative tells her that apparently a glitch in the computer's software caused the unexpected results. He tells Jennifer that it is not likely to occur again but he cannot be totally sure.

What should Jennifer do?
Should the PFT procedure be classified as experimental?
Record your conclusions below:

_____
_____
_____
_____
_____
_____
_____
_____
_____

## STUDY QUESTIONS

1. Prepare a pro-and-con discussion on the following statement: "Human experimentation in health care occurs only when there is a carefully designed study with the stated purpose of proving or disproving a hypothesis."

2. List the three ethical principles that must be considered when human experimentation occurs. Briefly describe the significance of each.

3. Briefly contrast the difference between common practice and experimental care.

4. Identify procedures in respiratory care where the line between common practice and experimental care is blurred.

## REFERENCES

1. Brandt, M: Racism and research: The case of the Tuskegee syphilis study. Hastings Center Report 8(6):21–29, December 1978.
2. Biomedical ethics and the shadow of nazism: A conference on the proper use of the Nazi analogy in ethical debate, April 1976. Hastings Center Report 6(4): special supplement, August 1976.
3. Husted, GL, and Husted, JH: Ethical Decision Making in Nursing. Mosby Year Book, St Louis, 1991, p 48.
4. Annas, G, et al: The Rights of Doctors, Nurses and Allied Health Professionals. Ballinger, Cambridge, MA, 1981, p 131.

## ADDITIONAL SUGGESTED READINGS

1. Beauchamp, TL, and Childress, JF: Principles of Biomedical Ethics, ed 3. Oxford University Press, New York, 1989.
2. Ellos, WJ: Patients' rights. In Monagle, JF, and Thomasma, D (Eds): Medical Ethics: A Guide for Health Professionals. Aspen Publishers, Rockville, MD, 1988, pp 317–323.
3. Capron, AM: Human experimentation. In Veatch, RM (Ed): Medical Ethics. Jones and Bartlett, Boston, 1989, pp 125–172.
4. Beauchamp, T: Informed consent. In Veatch, RM (Ed): Medical Ethics. Jones and Bartlett, Boston, 1989, pp 173–200.
5. Walters, L: Genetics and reproductive technologies. In Veatch, RM (Ed): Medical Ethics. Jones and Bartlett, Boston, 1989, pp 201–219.

# CHAPTER 10

# *Dealing With Difficult Patients*

**The Issue**
The Noncompliant Patient
Patients Who Demand Extraordinary Attention
Patients Who Violate Hospital Rules
"Undesirables"
Patient-Centered Care

**Legal Considerations**
**Ethical Considerations**
**Therapeutic Communication**
**Case Study**
Case Study 9

## THE ISSUE

Inevitably, in the process of delivering care, the health care practitioner is likely to encounter patients with whom the practitioner's interaction will be less than optimal due to the patient's behavior, attitude, or demeanor. Health care practitioners might also find that their own behavior, attitude, or demeanor may be affected by preconceived notions about some of the patients with whom they interact. These patients constitute what health care practitioners generally refer to as "difficult" patients. Difficult patients pose a dilemma for the health care provider since it is a general belief that a positive rapport with the patient is essential to good care. The issue of difficult patients is covered in a textbook on legal and ethical dilemmas since practitioners' attitudes and actions and their ability to make appropriate decisions may be affected when patients are deemed to be difficult.

When confronted with a difficult patient, regardless of the reason, health care providers often find themselves reexamining their personal values as well as the ethical principles routinely used for decision making. In some cases, they may attempt to avoid the patient since it is human nature to avoid difficult situations. Other typical reactions include an eye-for-an-eye attitude or outright revenge if the health care practitioner believes that the patient is purposely being difficult. Of course, revengeful behavior will generally be denied by most health care providers. Obviously, none of these human reactions is an appropriate way of dealing with patients when the objective is to provide the best possible care.

Even though there is no precise definition of what really constitutes a difficult patient, these patients fall into several general categories. The most common category is probably the noncompliant, or nonconforming, patient. Noncompliance may be related to many things including fear or discomfort on the part of the patient. Other categories include patients who demand disproportionate attention and patients who violate hospital rules. The final category of difficult patients includes those whom the health care practitioner may perceive as difficult simply because they are different or because they engage in behavior that the health care practitioner considers to be substandard or immoral. These patients are often thought of as simply being "undesirables." A brief discussion of types of difficult patients follows.

## The Noncompliant Patient

A major underlying premise of the delivery of health care is the assumption that patients will comply, in most cases, without question, with the directions and recommendations of health care providers. When working with a noncompliant patient, health care practitioners may feel that their role of delivering good care is being challenged by the patient.[1] Actually, patients may refuse to cooperate for many different reasons. As stated earlier, common reasons include fear and discomfort. The health care environment is a totally new experience for most patients; they have only a vague idea of what to expect. This experience comes at a time when the patient is either suffering from pain or having concerns about his or her future well-being, or both. Many patients encountered by respiratory care practitioners will be experiencing shortness of breath and will be extremely frightened that very soon they will not be able to breathe. Table 10–1 contains some common reasons for patients' noncompliance.

It is important for the health care practitioner to keep in mind that lack of compliance on the part of patients is not necessarily intentional. Patients may assume that they are complying; however, they may not clearly understand the wishes of the health care practitioner. Some patients may also be simply engaged in a subconscious strategy to reduce their fear by ensuring continuous attention from the health care practitioners. The noncompliant patient presents a critical dilemma for the health care practitioner. In order for the therapeutic process to work and lead to wellness, the patient must comply with the treatment process. But, if the patient does not believe that the therapeutic process will work, he or she is in a position to create a self-fulfilling prophecy. In this case, the patient's reason for not complying is reinforced by his or her own noncompliance. Some specific suggestions on dealing with noncompliant patients are offered later in this chapter.

Table 10–1. COMMON REASONS FOR THE PATIENTS' NONCOMPLIANCE

- Fear
  of the unknown
  of pain
  of appearing unintelligent
  of surrendering control of the body to strangers
  of a diagnosis
  of the prognosis
- Discomfort
  associated with pain
  associated with unfamiliar surroundings
  associated with unfamiliar people and procedures
- Lack of understanding concerning what the patient should do to comply

## Patients Who Demand Extraordinary Attention

These patients routinely expect and demand a level of attention that surpasses that needed for quality care for their condition. These patients can be particularly frustrating to the health care practitioner since one of the goals of health care is to provide quality care to all patients. Quality of care and level of care, however, are not necessarily equivalent.

*Quality of care* is generally defined by the health care practitioner as the delivery of needed care at a standard consistent with what other professionals would deliver or with whatever would be expected by the community. *Level of care* relates to the intensity and frequency with which care is provided to the patient. Patients sometimes confuse these two concepts and assume that in order to ensure quality care, they must receive continuous attention. Only the health care practitioner, using his or her professional judgment and the orders of the attending physician, can make the appropriate decisions about the level and amount of care to deliver to each patient. Some patients, however, will not accept this and will constantly demand attention. Sometimes, this type of behavior on the part of the patient is also caused by fear of the unknown. The health care practitioner must remember in these cases that, although it is not possible to give all patients all the time they desire, it is essential that all contacts with patients exhibit respect and quality care.[2]

## Patients Who Violate Hospital Rules

Hospitals and other health care institutions must operate within a clear set of rules to ensure the well-being of all patients. For example, visiting hours are generally limited. Visitors under a certain age, for example, children under 12 years old, may not be allowed. The number of visitors that a patient may have at one time may be limited. Patients and visitors are generally banned from smoking or drinking alcohol. A patient may be prohibited from eating certain foods. Drugs that a patient may have been taking at home will generally also be banned. These rules are usually detailed in a brochure given to the patient or family members upon admission. These rules are not arbitrary but are designed to ensure the smooth operation of the institution. Patients who refuse to comply with the rules of the institution place their well-being and the well-being of other patients in jeopardy.

## "Undesirables"

This category of difficult patients is probably the most difficult to pin down. The reason for this is that although health care practitioners may see these patients as undesirables, their training may have conditioned them not to admit their true feelings. Part of the difficulty in describing these patients is based on the subjective interpretation of the facts associated with the behavior or situation that leads the health care practitioner to apply the undesirable label. Such patients' behavior or situation may be legal or illegal. For example, patients may be viewed negatively because they have a lifestyle that varies from the community norm or because they have been convicted of a heinous crime. The latter example is clearly illegal behavior, whereas one's lifestyle, generally, is not a legal issue. The undesirable label also may be simply a matter of judgment on the part of the health care practitioner based on his or her own personal values. Consciously or subconsciously, health care practitioners may judge certain behaviors or situations on a continuum ranging from simply being substandard to completely immoral. Their interactions with patients will be affected by their judgment.

Patients from slum neighborhoods where minimal preventive health care is practiced may be preconceived as undesirable simply because their state of health is poor or because they seem to show little motivation to change. Of course, there is nothing illegal about this type of behavior or situation. In contrast, patients from more up-scale neighborhoods may be viewed more favorably even though they are involved in substance abuse, and yet their behavior is clearly illegal. Some health care practitioners may also have difficulty dealing with patients who are hospitalized with complications associated with legal abortion or attempted suicide. Without a doubt, health care practitioners are entitled to have personal views and moral standards; however, they may create ethical dilemmas for themselves when they begin to apply their personal views to their patients. The following exercise may assist the practitioner in sorting out feelings concerning undesirable patients.

## APPLIED EXERCISE 10-1

Sally W. is a 35-year-old divorced woman. She has had five children by three different fathers and is currently pregnant. Five years ago she was addicted to drugs and engaged in various illegal activities to support her habit. She is now hospitalized following a suicide attempt after an unsuccessful effort to abort her current pregnancy. In addition to her history, Sally is uncooperative and appears not to be concerned about her progress.

1. List the behaviors/situations that might be used by some health care practitioners to classify Sally as an undesirable patient.

_____

_____

_____

2. Classify these behaviors as legal or illegal.
3. How else might these behaviors be classified?
4. To what extent should the health care practitioner allow the patient's previous or current behaviors to influence the care delivered to the patient?

## Patient-Centered Care

One very interesting group of patients that are sometimes considered by health care providers to be difficult may in fact be part of an emerging trend that can be described as patient-centered care. Patient-centered care differs significantly from patient-focused care, another concept currently popular in health care circles. Whereas patient-focused care deals with the concentration of resources around each patient with the patient remaining relatively passive, patient-centered care deals with highly motivated patients who, in addition to assuming responsibility for their own care, insist on being active in the decision-making process surrounding their care. These patients:

- Do not hesitate to disagree with their health advisors
- Frequently choose to explore alternative holistic therapies
- Have an awareness of tremendous cost of health care
- Have an awareness of hazards as well as potential benefits of health care
- Seek second, third, fourth, etc., opinions if they feel the need
- Refuse to become victims, regardless of the disease
- Demand dignity, personhood, and control, regardless of the disease

Unfortunately, the characteristics of this type of patient may often be labeled as difficult by health care providers.[3]

## LEGAL CONSIDERATIONS

Legal considerations in dealing with difficult patients relate primarily to the need to provide the same standard of care to difficult patients as would be provided to other patients. Failure to do so may result in charges of malpractice, leaving both the practitioner and the institution liable for damages. Disapproval of the patient's behavior, attitude, or lifestyle is not a legitimate reason for denying the patient the highest possible standard of care. A review of Chapter 2 may refresh the reader's memory about potential legal complications associated with treating these patients differently than other patients.

## ETHICAL CONSIDERATIONS

The overriding ethical principle when dealing with difficult patients is the principle of justice. Simply stated, the difficult patient must receive the maximum care to which he or she is entitled. The care should be delivered without regard to any label imposed on the patient. In addition to the principle of justice, all the other ethical principles apply as appropriate. For example, these patients are still entitled to autonomy, beneficence, fidelity, veracity, and confidentiality.

There is no one best way of dealing with difficult patients since each situation is different. However, the guidelines in Box 10-1 may assist health care practitioners in devising a positive approach to these patients.

## THERAPEUTIC COMMUNICATION

One way of enhancing communication with all patients, including difficult ones, is to employ therapeutic communication as much as possible. There is no precise definition for therapeutic communication. However, as the name implies, the objective is to communicate in such a way that the effectiveness of the practitioner-patient interaction is maximized. Therapeutic communication does not involve engaging in psychotherapy with the patient. As with effective communication in general, therapeutic communication has certain essential elements. Some of the most important elements are listed and summarized below.

- *Acknowledgement of the patient as a person.* Interactions in which the patient is treated as a nonbeing or as an objective that must be cared for will decrease the

---

**Box 10-1. GENERAL "RULES" FOR DEALING WITH DIFFICULT PATIENTS**

1. Maintain a professional attitude at all times while treating the "difficult" patient, the same as you would for any other patient.
2. Maintain a positive attitude at all times while focusing on delivering care with the greatest skill and integrity possible.
3. Do not allow the patient's behavior, attitude, or demeanor to influence the quality or level of care being delivered.
4. Communicate as much information to the patient as possible about his or her care, the frequency of your visits, and the time when you will return. The purpose of the therapy and the procedures should always explained clearly to the patient. The patient should be given the opportunity to ask questions.
5. Treat the patient with dignity, care, and concern.

patient's respect for the care giver. It may also decrease the patient's trust and confidence in the process. Acknowledging the patient as a person involves calling the patient by name, making and maintaining appropriate eye contact with the patient, and taking some interest in the patient beyond his or her illness.

- *Use active and reflective listening.* Active listening involves what you do with both your ears and your body. You not only listen with your ears but show that you are listening with your body language. Do not turn your back or continue to busily perform some task while the patient is talking. Reflective listening involves repeating or summarizing some of the things the patient has said as a way of clarifying and verifying that you heard what the patient said.
- *Focus on the patient's concerns.* Respond to concerns expressed by the patient. In addition to responding to direct questions, you should also acknowledge and respond to any nuances that may be apparent in what the patient says. For example, if the patient implies that he or she is afraid of dying by saying, "I doubt I will see another summer," acknowledge that you understand that the patient is experiencing fear.
- *Keep the conversation positive.* Focus on the positive things happening to the patient. Although you do not want to give the patient false hope, there is no therapeutic value in engaging in a gloom-and-doom conversation with the patient.

These elements, although not inclusive of all that occurs in therapeutic communication, will be helpful to the respiratory care practitioner when engaging in verbal interactions with patients.

## CASE STUDY

### Case Study 9

Sandy R. is a registered therapist in a 225-bed community hospital in a medium-size town. At the start of the evening shift, she receives a report on a new patient who is in the intensive care unit. The patient has been hospitalized secondary to complications of an illicit drug overdose. The therapist giving the report refers to the patient as "a street person who is just taking up intensive care space." Sandy does not respond to her coworker's comment; however, she visualizes the patient as being somewhat undesirable. The patient is critically ill and is on continuous mechanical ventilation. Following the report, Sandy goes to the unit to check on her assigned patients. At this point, she recognizes the ventilator patient discussed in the report as old high school classmate. Her first reaction is anger that slowly turns to disgust as she performs her assessment of the patient.

1. What are the key legal issues?
2. What are the key ethical issues?
3. Who has rights in this case and what are they?
4. What are the responsibilities of the health care practitioners?

## STUDY QUESTIONS

1. *The following two patients are brought into the emergency room at the same time:*
   Patient A: *This patient is a police officer who has been allegedly shot by a man who the officer was attempting to apprehend after the officer entered the man's house to arrest him on a drug charge.*
   Patient B: *This patient is the man who allegedly shot patient A (the police officer) and who was subsequently shot by the officer's partner.*
   - Which of these patients should receive priority assuming both injuries appear to be similar?

   - Do you think the treatment decisions for either patient will be influenced by their status?

   - Is one of these patients likely to be labeled undesirable? If so, why?

2. *When a patient behaves in a difficult manner because of fear, what can the health care practitioner do to assist in allaying this fear?*

3. *What are some of the personal values held by a health care practitioner that may influence his or her interactions with difficult patients?*

## REFERENCES

1. Purtilo, R: Ethical Dimensions in the Health Professions, ed. 2. Saunders, Philadelphia, 1993, p 143.
2. Navarra, T, et al: Therapeutic Communication: A Guide to Effective Interpersonal Skills for Health Care Professionals. Slack Inc., Thorofare, NJ, 1990, p 78.
3. Ferguson, T: Patient, heal thyself: Health in the information age. The Futurist, January–February 1992, pp 9–13.

# CHAPTER 11

*Caring for Patients with Chronic Illnesses or Communicable Diseases*

> The Issue
> Patients With Chronic Illnesses
> Patients With Communicable Diseases
> **Legal Considerations**
> **Ethical Considerations**
> **Guidelines for Delivery of Care**
> **Case Studies**
> Case Study 10
> Case Study 11

## THE ISSUE

Both chronically ill patients and those with communicable diseases present unique challenges to the respiratory care practitioner. Chronically ill patients often make very little progress, and the prognosis for these patients is often poor. Under these frustrating circumstances, practitioners often become discouraged and distressed. In the case of patients with communicable diseases, practitioners are likely to experience considerable distress to the extent of fear for their own health. As a result, health care practitioners may experience a decrease not only in productivity but in the ability to maintain their own health. The ability to make rational legal and ethical decisions may be compromised. For these reasons, the practitioner must be aware of the profound personal impact of caring for these patients. Further, the practitioner must remember that regardless of any personal distress, the obligation to provide the highest level of care possible to these patients remains.

What are some of the reasons for distress associated with caring for patients with chronic conditions or communicable diseases? As a group, health care practitioners usually have healing as their goal. Since chronically ill patients do not improve, the resultant frustration on the part of the practitioner may lead to feelings of inadequacy, and such negative feelings toward performing a job are a common workplace stressor.[1]

Worry is another major stressor. In a 1990 study designed to identify stigmata related to AIDS and homophobia, it was concluded that AIDS is seen more as a value-laden human condition than as a medical condition caused by a virus.[2] However, a follow-up study in 1993 concluded that major concerns among nurses caring for HIV-positive persons included significant worry about contracting the virus and passing it on to their families. Nevertheless, this same study revealed a strong commitment to providing care to HIV/AIDS patients within the limits of professional expectations.[3]

Stress researchers have established that worry interferes with performance.[4] Prolonged worry leads to burnout and declining performance. Poor performance not only may result in poor patient care but may also endanger the health of the health care practitioner. Thus, it is important for the practitioner to recognize and develop coping mechanisms for dealing with patient populations such as those with chronic or communicable diseases.

## Patients With Chronic Illnesses

The most common chronic condition treated by respiratory care practitioners is chronic obstructive pulmonary disease (COPD). Since the major cause of COPD is smoking, this disease is largely viewed as a preventable condition. Some practitioners, therefore, may be less than positive about providing care to these patients, raising the ethical dilemma of whether it is appropriate to treat patients differently because they have a preventable disease. Other relatively common chronic conditions encountered by respiratory care practitioners are cystic fibrosis, interstitial lung disease, and asthma.

## Patients With Communicable Diseases

Today's health care practitioner is faced with caring for patients with a wide variety of communicable diseases. Many of these diseases are life-threatening for the patient and potentially dangerous for the health care practitioner. The health care practitioner has reason to be concerned about communicable diseases since these diseases have had a major impact on the lives of many. Diseases such as plague, leprosy, smallpox, and malaria have in some cases altered the direction of entire civilizations. The diseases of most concern currently include the human immunodeficiency virus (HIV), hepatitis B, and drug-resistant tuberculosis. With proper education and proper precautions, the health care provider faces only minimal risk from these diseases; however, the actual risk may be distorted by the common public perception of the risk involved.

The most controversial disease in this category is acquired immunodeficiency syndrome (AIDS). AIDS was first discussed in the medical literature in the early 1980s. At first, AIDS was described primarily as a disease of homosexuals. In fact, one of the early names assigned to the disease was gay related immunodeficiency disease (GRID). This labeling was probably one of the most unfortunate events in the history of HIV/AIDS. The association of the disease with homosexuality led many to view this strange new disease as something that the average person did not have to worry about. It also set the stage for potential discrimination against homosexual individuals and created many major ethical dilemmas. In fact, the view that AIDS is strictly a disease that affects homosexuals is misguided. The disease is nondiscriminatory and attacks without regard to sexual orientation, age, or social status.

Fortunately, despite the views of some individuals, HIV/AIDS is now accepted to be a serious health care problem to the general population. As with all communicable diseases there is some risk to the health care practitioner who provides care to the HIV/AIDS patient. The Centers for Disease Control and the Occupational Safety and Health Administration Agency have developed comprehensive procedures to protect health care providers as well as others who may be placed at risk through work activities. It is every health care practitioner's legal and ethical responsibility to follow all precautions for the effective prevention of transmitting HIV.

Concurrent with the increased awareness of danger from body fluids associated with the human immunodeficiency virus, new attention has been focused on the dangers of health care workers contracting hepatitis B. In fact, most health care workers are aware that hepatitis B may pose a threat at least equal to HIV. In 1993, it was estimated that over 300,000 people were infected with hepatitis B; however, only 12,000 of these cases were reported.[5]

## LEGAL CONSIDERATIONS

Like many other situations, the primary legal consideration associated with dealing with chronically ill patients or patients with communicable diseases relates primarily to the need to provide the same standard of care to these patients as would be provided to any other patients. Generally, practitioners may not refuse to treat patients simply because of their diagnosis. The one exception to this might be the situation in which the practitioner's fear is so strong that it may interfere with the care provided to the patient. Each hospital will have policy statements that clarify the practitioner's rights and obligations in these types of cases.

## ETHICAL CONSIDERATIONS

Several major ethical principles are associated with caring for chronically ill patients and patients with communicable diseases. They include autonomy, justice, the duty to not inflict injury or harm (nonmaleficence), and the duty to be faithful (fidelity). Simply stated, the practitioner cannot ethically treat this type of patient in any way different from the way he or she treats other patients. The fact that the patient's prognosis is at best bleak does not take away the patient's right to make decisions for himself or herself. Nor does it in any way give the practitioner the green light for providing less than optimal care.

## GUIDELINES FOR DELIVERY OF CARE

In spite of the nature of the patient's illness, a preventable chronic condition or a condition that might pose some danger to the practitioner, the obligation to deliver the best possible care remains.

- *The delivery of therapy should meet the highest level of excellence possible within prescribed standards of care.* This guideline may lead the practitioner to modify the standard of care to conform to the patient's need; however, the level of excellence used to deliver the care should not be compromised. For example, a patient may not be able or may not desire to complete an aerosol treatment. It would be appropriate for the practitioner to comply with the patient's desire in this case; however, it would not be appropriate for the practitioner to take the attitude that the treatment should be omitted altogether because "the patient isn't going to make it anyway."
- *Goals of care must take into consideration the patient's condition and the patient's understanding of his or her condition.* Goals of care for respiratory care practitioners usually involve some progressive improvement in pulmonary function. It may be inappropriate to set such a goal for the chronically ill COPD patient. The care goal may be simply to provide quality care to a level of comfort defined by the patient.
- *Consideration must be given to the patient's need to modify the therapy to fit into any lifestyle changes caused by the chronic condition or contagious disease.* In the case of chronic conditions like COPD, patients may need to adapt their activities of daily living in a way that allows them to maximize their energy. Since the objective of therapy in this case is not to cure the condition, but to bring the highest level of comfort possible to the patient, the practitioner should be willing to modify therapy as much as possible to assist the patient in reaching his or her goal. In the case of contagious diseases, the patient may have concerns about accidentally transmitting the disease to others. The practitioner should be cognitive of this.
- *Practitioners must protect themselves both from the stress involved as well as from any physical danger.* Patient care always carries with it a relatively high level of distress. Caring for patients with chronic or contagious diseases is likely to intensify the distress experienced by the practitioner. The practitioner should not hesitate to seek appropriate relief from distress. Appropriate time off, opportunities for relaxation, and effective time management are

all things that should be considered in an ongoing stress reduction program. Practitioners should also take all the appropriate precautions to protect themselves from contracting any contagious diseases carried by the patient. This should be done in a routine and matter-of-fact manner.

##  APPLIED ACTIVITY 11–1

This chapter illustrates the importance of avoiding or reducing distress as an important part of being able to make rational legal and ethical decisions. Certain stress management tools are available that many people have found to be useful. Among them are:
- Time management
- The relaxation response
- Positive affirmations
- Emotional diversification
- Physical exercise

Select one of the tools that you think might be effective for you. Using library or other available resources, write a one- or two-page paper on how this tool works and how you might use it.

## CASE STUDIES

### Case Study 10

> At age 21, Katy had it all. She was beautiful and full of life. A university junior, she was 1 year from graduation. Life was wonderful for Katy, that is, until she was involved in an auto accident that left her paralyzed for life. Since the accident, she not only suffers from the trauma of paralysis but her body is also weakened by chronic kidney failure and recurrent infections. Realistically, she is not likely to live very long. Katy's parents, upset that their daughter is being taken away, insist on having "everything possible" done for her. Katy, who is mentally alert most of the time, endures on a daily basis hours of therapy. She complains to everyone who will listen: her physician, her nurses, her physical and respiratory therapist. She wants to die and insists that existing like this is not living. With each passing week, Katy loses weight and grows weaker. Her parents become angry whenever they hear these comments from Katy, and they insist that the care providers "do all they can."

1. What are the key legal issues?
2. What are the key ethical issues?
3. What are Katy's rights?
4. What are Katy's parents' rights?
5. What are the responsibilities of the health care practitioners?

## Case Study 11

John's job as the chief executive officer of a massive health care complex often gave him headaches. He assumed the headaches were simply caused by stress—the price one paid for being CEO. One afternoon after a particularly difficult day, John's headache becomes so unbearable that he passes out. He is admitted to his own hospital and diagnosed as having had a massive stroke. He falls into a coma and his prognosis is considered grave. It is expected that he will die within a few days to a week. The best medical technology available in the hospital is provided for him.

John's wife, aware that he has a living will stating that "extraordinary procedures" are not to be performed, hesitates to call attention to the living will. She rationalizes that the end is near, and so why rush it. John, however, lingers on in a vegetative state. After several months, it becomes clear that although he is not improving, death is not imminent. John's new prognosis is that he may live in this state for years. John's wife decides to attempt to have the living will provisions implemented. Since she had waited, several legal questions arise and a hearing is scheduled to determine whether the document is binding and should be honored. The day before the scheduled hearing, John awakens from the coma. After a few days, he has a new prognosis. Now his doctors expect him to have some short-term memory loss and mild physical weakness on one side of his body, but otherwise they expect him to be fine. John recovers and goes home.

Five years later, John is living a quiet life doing medical management consulting out of his home. After progressively losing weight and several bouts of pneumonia, John is diagnosed as having full-blown AIDS. As best as can be determined, the virus was contracted during the previous hospital stay. John's wife is also HIV-positive. He is again admitted to the hospital where he had worked previously. Within a very short time following his admission, John's diagnosis becomes common knowledge among the hospital staff.

Jan is a new respiratory care practitioner at the hospital. She is 23 years old, and recently married. When she is assigned to deliver aerosol treatments to John, she requests that someone else deliver the treatment since she is attempting to get pregnant. The supervisor attempts to accommodate Jan, but all the other staff members also refuse saying that Jan cannot select to treat only the patients she prefers. All the other staff members have at other times treated patients with AIDS.

1. What are the key legal issues?
2. What are the key ethical issues?

3. What are Jan's rights?
4. What are the rights and responsibilities of the health care practitioners in this case?

## STUDY QUESTIONS

1. Why might health care practitioners find it frustrating to care for patients who are chronically ill?

2. In what ways is it acceptable to provide a different level of care for a patient who is chronically ill as opposed to a patient who is not?

3. When might it be acceptable for a specific practitioner to request to be relieved from treating a patient with a communicable disease?

4. What are some of the stress management practices health care practitioners should engage in to ensure that they can effectively care for chronically ill patients and patients with communicable diseases?

5. What is the relationship between distress and work performance?

6. What major ethical principle was clearly violated in Case Study 10?

## REFERENCES

1. Byer, CO, and Shainberg, LW: Living Well: Health Is Your Hands, ed 2. HarperCollins, New York, 1995, p 85.
2. Wright, B, and Yates, RB: AIDS and homophobia: A perspective for AIDS educators. Feminist Teacher 1990; 4:10–12.

3. Laschinger, HKS, and Goldenberg, D: Attitudes of practicing nurses as predictors of intended care behavior with persons who are HIV positive: Testing the Ajzen-Fishbein theory of reasoned action. Research in Nursing and Health 1993; 16: 441–450.
4. Smith, JC: Understanding Stress and Coping. Macmillan, New York, 1993, p 199.
5. Centers for Disease Control: Cases of selected notifiable diseases, United States, weeks ending December 25, 1993, and December 19, 1992 (51th week), MMWR 42(51 & 52): 998–1,000, January 7, 1994.

## ADDITIONAL SUGGESTED READINGS

1. Carroll, C: Stress: Prevention and Control Strategies for Health Care Professionals. Educational Resources Consortium, Claremont, CA, 1992.

# CHAPTER 12

# *Caring for the Terminally Ill and Dying Patient*

**The Issue**
The Terminally Ill Patient
The Dying Patient
**Legal Considerations**
Death Protocols

**Ethical Considerations**
Patients' Right to Know
Appropriate Treatment for the Dying Person
**Case Study**
Case Study 12

## THE ISSUE

Cardiopulmonary resuscitation and managing life support systems are two major components of modern respiratory care. Respiratory care practitioners take great pride in their ability to resuscitate patients, intubate and manage them on ventilators, and wean them from the equipment. These procedures bring needed relief from respiratory distress to many patients and allow them to resume their daily routines after recuperating from otherwise life-threatening illness. When performing these procedures for patients who recover, the practitioner is certainly performing his or her duties within the framework of the ethical principle of beneficence.

In many cases, however, even though the practitioner adeptly performs resuscitation and life support management procedures, it becomes clear that the patient will never leave the hospital and in some cases that the patient will never be disconnected from the life support equipment. Thus, the intended benefit to patients does not occur, and perhaps the practitioner's procedures may be at odds with the principle of nonmaleficence—not to inflict harm on patients. This dilemma has existed ever since modern medicine developed the capability of prolonging clinical life. And as more equipment and advanced procedures become available, this dilemma will become more common and complex.

Caring for the terminally ill patient presents modern health care practitioners with a challenging ethical dilemma. Medical health care currently focuses on using new technology and advanced drug therapy to heal and improve the quality of life for humankind. Thus, when the reality of death enters the equation, health care workers are sometimes unsure as to what their role should be. This confusion has been heightened by additional questions concerning the allocation of resources and accessibility of care for everyone. Inherent in the philosophy of the medical model of health care is the dictum that every effort should be made to heal the patient up until the last possible moment before death. The ethical dilemma centers on the following challenging questions: Who is terminally ill? Can it be known whether a patient is terminally ill prior to death, or is it only a way of classifying patients retrospectively? How much care should be given while the patient is terminally ill? Should available resources be saved for patients who are not terminally ill?

Health care practitioners must work with many different types of terminally ill patients—those with various forms of cancer or end-stage organ failure due to a variety of causes and victims of accidents. Some terminal illnesses are chronic in nature. Respiratory care practitioners routinely deal with one of the most common chronic and ultimately terminal diseases: chronic obstructive lung disease.

## The Terminally Ill Patient

In this era of modern medical technology, which has the capability to support vital organ function, it is not easy to define death. It is even more difficult to define terminal illness. Death implies a finale, an end point. Terminal illness on other hand, implies a process that will ultimately result in death. The difficulty with this definition is that it is impossible to predict with any accuracy if and when a patient will die.

Guidelines have been designed to show the practitioner how to treat terminally ill patients as well as to help determine when death has occurred. One set of guidelines was developed by Massachusetts General Hospital. Titled "Guidelines for Optimum Care of the Critically Ill," they first appeared in the *New England Journal of Medicine* in 1976.[1] The guidelines are summarized here (Box 12–1), not because they outline a "correct" system, but because they are representative of a good system.

Part of the dilemma about the type of care to be provided is related to the location in which care will be provided. Terminally ill patients are usually housed in the hospital, in an extended care facility (nursing home, etc.), or at home. Hospice care, which is rapidly becoming a part of providing care for the dying, may be a part of any of these settings. There are advantages and disadvantages to each of these settings. Also, to some degree, the legal and ethical considerations change with each setting since by choosing the setting, the patient or the person responsible for the patient's care is consciously accepting and rejecting certain choices for that patient.

Hospice care is more of a concept than a specific location. Hospice care may simply be a team approach to care (regardless of the patient's location), it may be a

> **Box 12–1. SUMMARY OF THE ESSENTIAL COMPONENTS OF GUIDELINES FOR OPTIMUM CARE OF THE CRITICALLY ILL**
>
> Whenever appropriate, critically ill patients should be classified according to the level of care needed.
>
> Level 1
>
> This level is for patients with a good prognosis. Maximal therapeutic care should be delivered.
>
> Level 2
>
> This level is for patients with an unclear prognosis. Maximal therapeutic care should be delivered; however, the patient's prognosis should be regularly evaluated to determine if the correct level is assigned.
>
> Level 3
>
> This level is for patients with a poor prognosis. Therapeutic care should be delivered on a selective basis. The primary considerations should be to maintain patient comfort as well as to limit or stop the progression of the patient's illness to the extent possible.
>
> Level 4
>
> This level is for patients with an extremely poor prognosis. Care should be for comfort purposes as opposed to therapeutic purposes.

specific unit in a hospital, or it may be a free-standing unit. For the most part, "hospice" in the United States refers to an interdisciplinary support network of care givers who care for patients dying at home. The National Hospice Organization defines hospice care as "a medically directed, interdisciplinary program of palliative services for terminally ill people and their families."[2] It is easy to see that within the hospice definition the major goals are patient and family comfort and emotional support.

The hospital is one of the locations in which respiratory care practitioners are highly likely to provide care for the terminally ill patient. Therapy for the patient in the hospital setting may involve critical care life support or simply palliative care to reduce suffering. The latter instance is most likely to provide difficulty for the respiratory care practitioner, since therapists are trained to believe that good therapy should result in progressive improvement of the patient's health status. When terminally ill patients are in the hospital, they are usually there either because they were hospitalized prior to the terminally ill prognosis or because they need specialized supportive care that can only be provided in a hospital setting.

Since extended care facilities are being used more frequently, respiratory care practitioners are also likely to encounter many terminally ill patients in these facilities. Many of these patients are also in need of supportive or palliative care. Practitioners who work in these settings may have less difficulty dealing with the nature of terminal care simply because it may be more consistent with the kind of care they routinely provide.

Regardless of the location of care, it is important for the respiratory care practitioner to realize that therapy for terminally ill patients, like therapy for all patients, should be delivered according to the guidelines listed below. It is no accident that these guidelines are similar to those listed in Chapter 11 for delivering care to patients with chronic illnesses or contagious diseases.

- *The delivery of therapy should meet the highest level of excellence possible within prescribed standards of care.* This guideline may lead the practitioner to modify the standard of care to conform to the patient's need; however, the level of excellence used to deliver care should not be compromised. For example, a patient may not be able or may not desire to complete an aerosol treatment. It would be appropriate for the practitioner to comply with the patient's desire in this case; however, the practitioner should not take the attitude that the treatment should be omitted altogether because "the patient isn't going to make it anyway."
- *Goals of care must take into consideration the patient's prognosis and the patient's understanding of his or her prognosis.* Goals of care for respiratory care practitioners usually involve some progressive improvement in pulmonary function. However, to set such a goal for the terminally ill patient may be inappropriate. The goal may be simply to provide quality care to a level of comfort defined by the patient.
- *Consideration must be given to the patient's need to bring closure, fulfillment, and satisfaction to other aspects of his or her life.* The patient's need to have visitors and to acknowledge and display cards and flowers may interfere with some aspects of his or her care. While certain rules and standards of care cannot and should not be compromised, it is extremely important for the practitioner to show compassion and understanding when the patient has these special needs.
- *Care must focus on the patient as a live person, not as a person who will soon be dead.* Although the patient's prognosis may indicate that the patient does not have much longer to live, the practitioner must remember that the patient is a living human and must be treated as such. The practitioner should be careful, in his or her choice of words and actions, not to imply that in a few days or weeks the patient might be dead. This should not be seen as contradictory to the need to modify care if necessary and to show compassion during the delivery of therapy.

## The Dying Patient

Death, as a final state, is easy to define. It is simply the permanent cessation of the function of the heart and lungs. This definition suffices when there is no interference with the function of the heart and lungs. Life support equipment, however, by its very definition is designed to support, either directly or indirectly, life's vital functions. Thus, a dilemma develops. It is sometimes difficult to determine whether there is a permanent cessation of heart and lung function when life support equipment is being used. However, since removing the patient from the equipment for a period of time to make this determination may subject the patient to irreversible damage, a criterion other than cessation of heart and lung function obviously must be used to define death. It also becomes obvious that defining death from a medical standpoint is not a simple task.

Harvard Medical School inadvertently took the lead in the efforts to redefine death by forming an ad hoc committee to develop a definition of irreversible coma. In 1968, when the committee presented its findings in an article in the *Journal of the American Medical Association* entitled "A Definition of Irreversible Coma," the word "coma" was inadvertently changed to "brain death." As a result, the committee's criteria, which was intended to define an irreversible coma, became the definition of brain death. The criteria included the following four conditions[3]:

1. *Unreceptivity and unresponsivity.* There is a total unawareness of externally applied stimuli and inner need and a complete unresponsiveness—our definition of irreversible coma. Even the most intensely painful stimuli evoke no vocal or other response, not even a groan, withdrawal of a limb, or quickening of respiration.

2. *No movements of breathing.* Observation by physicians covering a period of at least 1 hour is adequate to satisfy the criteria of no spontaneous muscular movements or spontaneous respirations or response to stimuli such as pain, touch, sound, or light. After the patient is on a mechanical ventilator, a total absence of spontaneous breathing may be established by turning off the ventilator for 3 minutes and observing whether the patient makes any effort to breathe spontaneously. (The ventilator may be turned off during this time provided that at the start of the trial period the patient's carbon dioxide tension is within the normal range and provided also that the patient had been breathing room air for at least 10 minutes prior to the trial.)

3. *No reflexes.* Irreversible coma with abolition of central nervous system activity is evidenced in part by the absence of elicitable reflexes. The pupil will be fixed and dilated and will not respond to a direct source of bright light. Since the establishment of a fixed, dilated pupil is clear-cut in clinical practice, there would be no uncertainty as to its presence. Ocular movement (to head turning and to irrigation of the ears with ice water) and blinking are absent. There is no evidence of postural activity (decerebrate or other). Swallowing, yawning, and vocalization are in abeyance. Corneal and pharyngeal reflexes are absent. As a rule the stretch of tendon reflexes cannot be elicited: that is, tapping the tendons of the biceps, triceps, and pronator muscles, quadriceps, and gastrocnemius muscles with the reflex hammer elicits no contraction of the respective muscles. Plantar and noxious stimulation elicit no response.

4. *Flat electroencephalogram (EEG).* Of great confirmatory value is the flat, or isoelectric, EEG. We must assume that the electrodes have been properly applied, that the apparatus is functioning normally, and that the personnel in charge are competent. We consider it prudent to have one channel of the ap-

paratus used for an electrocardiogram (ECG). This channel will monitor the ECG so that, if it appears in the electroencephalographic leads because of high resistance, it can be readily identified. It also established the presence of the active heart in the absence of the EEG. We recommend that another channel be used for a noncephalic lead to pick up space-borne or vibration-borne artifacts and identify them. The simplest form of such a monitoring noncephalic electrode has two leads over the dorsum of the hand, preferably the right hand, so that the ECG will be minimal or absent. Since one of the requirements of this state is that there be no muscle activity, these two dorsal hand electrodes will not be stimulated by muscle artifact. The apparatus should be run at standard gains 10 μV/mm, 50 μV/5mm. Also it should be isoelectric at double this standard gain which is 5 μV/mm or 25 μV/5mm. At least 10 full minutes of recording are desirable, but twice that would be better. It is also suggested that the gains at some point be opened to full amplitude for a brief period (5 to 100 seconds) to see what is going on. Usually, in an intensive care unit, artifacts dominate the picture, but these are readily identifiable. There should be no electroencephalographic response to noise or pinch.

All the above tests should be repeated at least 24 hours later with no change. The validity of such data as indications of irreversible cerebral damage depends on the exclusion of two conditions: hypothermia (temperature below 90°F [32.2°C] or the presence of central nervous system depressants, such as barbiturates.

Of course, the Harvard committee did not deliver the final word on brain death. In 1978, the Uniform Brain Death Act was developed in an attempt to clear up legal confusion concerning death. This act was refined with the Uniform Determination of Death Act in 1981.[4] The guidelines are included in Box 12–2.

A major issue associated with brain death is the "Do Not Resuscitate" (DNR) order. The DNR approach focuses not on defining death but rather on letting death take a natural course without intervention. The value of DNR orders is controversial and may be considered a moot issue among many practitioners. The fact is that cardiopulmonary resuscitation is successful only about one-third of the time and that only one-third of those successfully resuscitated actually leave the hospital alive.[4,5,6] The real value of the DNR order appears to lie in its contribution in allowing death to occur naturally in those cases where it is clearly imminent. DNR orders are now legal realities in many states with New York being the first to pass legislation to that effect.[6]

## LEGAL CONSIDERATIONS

Historically, the legal urgency to define death became apparent in 1968 when Kansas became the first state to pass a law permitting the procuring of organs for transplantation. It was immediately clear to physicians desiring to perform transplants that the traditional definition of cessation of function of the heart and lungs, used at that time, was an unworkable definition. Application of the traditional definition of death would damage the very organs intended for transplantation. Not all states immedi-

> **Box 12–2. GUIDELINES FOR THE DETERMINATION OF BRAIN DEATH**
>
> When the requirements of criteria 1, 2, and 3 are fulfilled, the patient may be pronounced brain dead by a licensed physician.
> 1. Coma of established irreversible cause or exclusion of reversible causes of coma. (a) The patient must have a known irreversible structural or systemic disease causing coma. (b) There must be no chance of drug intoxication or significant hypothermia (core temperature less than 33°C) contributing to the cause of coma. (c) A 6-hour period of observation during which tests of cerebral and brain stem function are performed and documented is sufficient when the nature and duration of coma are known. (d) Longer periods of observation and more testing may be necessary under some circumstances and when the nature and duration of coma are not known.
> 2. Absence of cerebral function. (a) There must be no behavioral or reflex response to noxious stimuli indicative of function above the level of the foramen magnum. (b) Although not a requirement, as isoelectroencephalogram (performed according to the criteria of the American EEG Society) for 30 minutes is confirmatory of brain death.
> 3. Absence of brain stem function. (a) The pupils must be fixed, unreactive to bright light. (b) There must be no oculovestibular response to 50-cc ice water caloric tests in both ears. (c) There must be apnea for 10 minutes during apneic oxygenation or when a $PaCO_2$ is greater than 60 mm Hg in the absence of metabolic alkalosis. These tests of absent breathing should be performed following hyperoxygenation on mechanical ventilation.

ately followed Kansas' lead, prompting the National Conference of Commissioners on Uniform State Laws to approve and recommend for enactment a Uniform Death Act in August 1978. While all states currently define death in some manner, it is amazing that for an event that will affect all of us, there is still considerable uncertainty as to which laws apply and how they will be applied. Dealing with death from a legal standpoint is still a complex task in our society.

## Death Protocols

Because of the complexity of dealing with death from a legal standpoint, some hospitals have established death protocols. These protocols serve as a step-by-step guide for practitioners to follow. Specific duties are assigned and responsibilities are defined. The protocols are valuable in that they reduce the distress associated with death experienced by the institution's staff and in some cases may even prevent legal complications. Box 12–3 contains a sample emergency department death protocol.

> **Box 12–3. SAMPLE EMERGENCY DEPARTMENT DEATH PROTOCOL FOR CHILDREN (MODIFIED FOR RESPIRATORY CARE PRACTITIONERS)**
>
> - A primary family liaison should be established for consistent communication. All medical information should flow between the established liaison and the attending physician.
> - The family should be made comfortable by placing them in a private room with refreshments and a telephone.
> - The family should have access to support services, for example, the clergy, key family members, and professional counselors as necessary.
> - If the parents are going to view the body, the treatment room should be restored to order. From a legal standpoint, it may be necessary to leave certain equipment attached to the body. Ask the attending physician for directions. The attending physician should be available to explain any tubes or other equipment still attached to the body. The parents may be encouraged to touch the child.
> - Ensure complete chart documentation.
> - It may be appropriate for the attending physician to approach the family about organ and tissue donation.

## ETHICAL CONSIDERATIONS

There is general agreement among ethicists that the right to die with dignity is probably the most important ethical issue for the dying. There are several aspects to the right to die with dignity ranging from the right of the patient to know the truth regarding appropriate treatment during the dying process to the patient's right to intervene and to control the dying process somewhat. There is some minor debate associated with the patient's right to know, whereas there is little debate about providing appropriate treatment during the dying process. There is major debate, however, about the patient's right to intervene in the dying process.

### Patients' Right to Know

Historically, there has been considerable debate over whether and when patients should be told that death is imminent. Part of the debate, of course, has dealt with the fact that it is not always easy to determine when death is imminent. The major part of the debate, however, was the belief that it was desirable to protect the patient from any unnecessary mental distress or suffering. It was believed that if the patient was informed of the strong likelihood of imminent death, the patient might lose all hope for recovery. These beliefs, rooted somewhat in the now-outdated ethical principle of paternalism, ignored the possibility that the patient might want to use his or her final days to prepare for death with dignity.

Opponents to the practice of withholding information from patients relied on the doctrine of informed consent. The doctrine, developed over the years in various ways including court cases, is now well entrenched in medical practice.[7] The essential components of this doctrine are listed in Box 12-4.

## Appropriate Treatment for the Dying Patient

Although the dying patient is entitled to a standard of care that is appropriate for his or her condition, many practitioners are uncomfortable treating a patient when it has been openly acknowledged that death is imminent. Following are some suggestions that will assist in interacting with the dying patient.

- *Always behave in an empathetic manner when dealing with the patient.* Behaving in an empathetic manner simply means that you make every effort to understand the patient's mood and viewpoint. It does not mean showing sympathy toward the patient.
- *Listen to the patient's thoughts and concerns.* Dying patients may have things that they need to say. In some cases, the patient will be asking for reassurance and comfort. If the practitioner engages in active listening, he or she will not need to respond to much of what the patient says. If a response is necessary, it should be straightforward and noninterfering. Do not lecture patients or give them false hope; however, do not display a "you are going to die and nothing matters" attitude.
- *Assist the patient in maintaining personal dignity.* This can be done by simply continuing to treat the patient as a person who has opinions, feelings, and desires. Give patients a choice whenever possible. Ask their opinion, and listen to their desires, when appropriate.

---

### Box 12-4. ESSENTIAL COMPONENTS OF THE DOCTRINE OF INFORMED CONSENT

In order for patients to make reasonable decisions concerning their own treatment, they must be given the following information:
- A thorough description of their present condition along with the associated risks of nontreatment.
- A description of the procedures involved in as well as the associated risks and benefits of any recommended treatment.
- A description of available alternatives to the recommended treatment.

**130**  *Applications and Practices*

The final ethical consideration, the patient's right to intervene in the dying process, will be dealt with in Chapter 13, Advanced Directives.

## ✓ APPLIED EXERCISE 12-1

In order to become comfortable with the dying process, the student might complete the following process: Read the obituary section of your local newspaper for several issues. Select two obituaries on the following basis: The first should be an obituary that elicited some discomfort while you were reading it. The second should be an obituary that you felt very comfortable reading. In the space below, spend a few minutes and briefly describe what you think each person's life might have been like.

**Obituary One:**

_____
_____
_____
_____

**Obituary Two:**

_____
_____
_____
_____

## CASE STUDY

### Case Study 12

> Blanche R. is an 84-year-old woman residing in an extended care facility that specializes in providing long-term ventilator support to unweanable patients. Blanche has been diagnosed with Alzheimer's disease and chronic obstructive lung disease. Her only living relative is her 62-year-old son, who is also in poor health. The son visits his mother daily and pays attention to every aspect of her care. He is devastated when his mother suffers a massive cerebral hemorrhage and sinks into a deep coma. His mother's physician, believing that she has suffered brain death, orders the appropriate test for determination. The test results confirm the physician's suspicions that Blanche is brain dead. The physician approaches the son about removing Blanche from the ventilator. The son protests and threatens to get a lawyer and file a lawsuit.

1. What are the key legal issues?
2. What are the key ethical issues?
3. What are Blanche's son's rights?
4. What are the hospital's rights?
5. What are the responsibilities of the health care practitioners?

## STUDY QUESTIONS

*1. Briefly summarize Harvard Medical School's efforts to define "brain death."*

*2. Briefly discuss the potential ethical dilemma that may arise when a patient is being declared dead with the expectations that his or her organs will be transplanted into another patient.*

*3. Why might "Do Not Resuscitate" orders be considered moot by some practitioners?*

*4. What are the major ethical issues associated with dealing with patients who have been informed that death is imminent?*

*5. What are the essential components of the Doctrine of Informed Consent?*

## REFERENCES

1. Massachusetts General Hospital Clinical Care Committee: Optimum care for hopelessly ill patients. N Engl Med 1976; (295): 362–364.
2. Stoddard, S: The Hospice Movement: A Better Way of Caring for the Dying. Vintage Books, New York, 1978, p 1.
3. Harvard Medical School, Ad Hoc Committee of the Harvard School to Examine the Definition of Brain Death: A definition of irreversible coma. JAMA 1968; (205): 337–340.

4. President's Commission for the Study of Ethical Problems in Medicine and Biomedical and Behavioral Research: Deciding to Forego Life-Sustaining Treatment. Washington, DC, 1983, pp 234–235.
5. Bedell, SE, Delbanco, TL, Cook, EF, and Epstein, FH: Survival after cardiopulmonary resuscitation in the hospital. N Engl J Med 1983; (309): 569–576.
6. Taffe, EG, Teasdale, TA, and Luchi, RJ: In-hospital cardiopulmonary resuscitation. Journal of the American Medical Association 1988; (260): 2069–2072.

# CHAPTER 13

# *Advance Directives*

**The Issue**
Ordinary Versus Extraordinary Care
**Legal Considerations**
Living Wills
Durable Power of Attorney for Health Care
Assisted-Suicide Activity
**Ethical Considerations**
**Case Study**
Case Study 13

## THE ISSUE

Consider the following patient population at City Memorial Hospital's five occupied beds in their 10-bed intensive care unit (ICU) on a recent Saturday morning:

*Bed 1*

John L. is attached to a Bennett 7200 ventilator. He is 85 years old and in late-stage emphysema. The decision to place him on the ventilator was made by his niece and nephew, his only living relatives. The niece and nephew are having breakfast in the hospital coffee shop and wondering what to do next. They ask each other, "Did Uncle John ever tell you his wishes about a situation like this?"

*Bed 2*

Carrie P. is on a pressure-assisted ventilator. She is only 46 but has suffered from pulmonary hypertension secondary to lupus erythematosus for the past 7 years, defying medical predictions that she would die within 2 or 3 years of her diagnosis. Her dream was to live until her son graduated from college. Her latest exacerbation started last week after returning from out of town where she had attended her son's graduation. She had been offered the opportunity to sign an advance directive but had refused to do so as long as her son was in college. Her son, dedicated to his mother for her emotional support in getting him through college, wants all that can be done for his mother to be done.

### Bed 3

(The ICU isolation room) Marvin A. is suffering from pneumocystis carinii pneumonia (PCP). Diagnosed as being HIV-positive 9 years ago, he is dying from AIDS. His mind is extremely foggy, but he does not want to be in the hospital. He also does not want to die alone.

### Bed 4

Bill W. is surrounded by a myriad of tubes and monitors. He is here as a result of a motorcycle spill a week earlier when he decided to take his bike for a quick spin to evaluate some repair work. The 19-year-old had figured that since he was only going around the block, he did not need to wear a helmet. He had never heard the term "advance directive." He had his first isoelectric EEG on Friday afternoon; the second one is scheduled for today. His parents are in the hospital coffee shop having breakfast and agonizing over the dilemma they face. At another time and place, Bill would have thought that the cyclic sounds of the ventilator augmented with various beeps and buzzes were cool. Now he is oblivious to them.

### Bed 5

Mildred P. was admitted following surgery yesterday. A single mother of six, she came to the hospital for an abdominal hysterectomy. However, after the procedure and as a result of her poorly treated hypertension, she suffered a cerebral vascular accident in recovery. The entire right side of her body is now paralyzed. She is semialert and wondering who is taking care of her kids.

The dilemma in all these cases is how to answer a simple question: How long should life be prolonged when the person is apparently terminally ill? The answer to this seemingly simple question is very complex. The issue of what to do when patients are terminally ill or simply do not want further treatment presents both an ethical and a legal dilemma. A major component of this dilemma is the quality-of-life issue. When asked casually, most of us will quickly answer that we no longer wish to live when our quality of life is gone. When asked to define what is meant by "quality of life," we immediately are challenged by the complexity of this concept.

Although there is no clear way to define quality of life, the following exercises should assist the reader in developing an appreciation of what is meant by the concept. There are two common ways of attempting to measure life's quality. The first is to focus on the physical state or capabilities of the body. Exercise 13–1 deals with this approach. The second way is to focus on mental capabilities or those things which make life enjoyable. Exercise 13–2 deals with this approach.

## ✓ APPLIED EXERCISE 13–1

Imagine that you as a healthy person begin to lose parts of your body, for example, a hand, an arm, or a leg, and so forth. How many body parts would you be willing to give up before your quality of life deteriorates to the point that you would rather be dead? Write your answer in the space below.

## ✓ APPLIED EXERCISE 13–2

On a single sheet of paper, make a list of the things which are mentally important to you and which you find fulfilling in life. Examples might include the ability to talk to others, to walk on the beach, and so on. When you complete the list, draw a line through each of the items that you are willing to give up before your quality of life deteriorates to the point that you would rather be dead. Make your list in the space below.

## Ordinary Versus Extraordinary Care

At the root of the discussion of advance directives is the debate concerning ordinary versus extraordinary care. As with many of the underlying issues in health care ethics, these terms are not easy to define. On the surface, it may appear that they can be defined on the basis of listing various advanced technological procedures and calling them extraordinary care. These advanced technological procedures would generally include those which prolong life artificially, implying that without these procedures, the patient would die. For respiratory care practitioners, the number one item on the list would be mechanical ventilation. During the 1960s and perhaps the

1970s, mechanical ventilation was clearly extraordinary care in the minds of most people. Is that still the case today? The answer is immediately less clear.

Other procedures that a decade or so ago may also have been considered extraordinary but today are somewhat routine include renal dialysis, basic and advanced cardiac resuscitation, open heart surgery, and selected drugs. Even procedures like heart transplants and reconnecting severed limbs are somewhat commonplace. It is clear that the line between ordinary and extraordinary care is quite blurred.

Who then should define extraordinary care, and how should it be defined? It appears that what is emerging is less a definition but more a matter of choice on the part of the patient. Patients, utilizing the various mechanisms afforded them through advance directives, are defining the level of care they wish to receive under various circumstances. Thus, regardless of whether mechanical ventilation is a form of extraordinary care, a patient may elect not to receive this type of care. The various advance directives mechanisms available to patients will be discussed later in this chapter. The utilization of advance directives is in no way a simple process, however, since there are still many legal and ethical hurdles that must be overcome.

## LEGAL CONSIDERATIONS

The legal issues associated with advance directives were brought to the forefront in a 1990 U.S. Supreme Court decision, *Missouri v. Cruzan,* in which the Court sent mixed signals. The Court decision recognized the constitutional right of competent patients to refuse medical treatment; however, the Court concluded that the regulation of these rights was to be based on state law. It was not a unanimous decision. Justice William Brennan wrote a strong dissenting opinion in which he kept alive the opinion that patients should be free from medical care without informed consent.[1] Justice Brennan's dissenting opinion was important in that it reemphasized the importance of informed consent. However, it did not help with one of the major problems with informed consent—the ultimate outcome of the procedure.

Of course, the opposing views associated with the decision created considerable confusion and controversy. In an attempt to resolve some of this confusion, Congress passed the federal Patient Self-Determination Act, which became effective in December of 1991.[2] The act requires that all health care facilities that receive reimbursement of Medicaid or Medicare funds must also inform their patients about their right to both refuse medical treatment and to sign advance directives. The act also prohibits health care providers from discriminating against individuals whether or not they sign advance directives. See Box 13–1 for specific provisions of the Act.

One of the main components of the Patient Self-Determination Act is the right of patients to execute advance directives. There are two types of advance directives: living wills and durable powers of attorney for health care. The purpose of advance directives is to give individuals a choice in medical decisions even when they may be unconscious or too ill to communicate. Advance directives are to be used only if patients are unable to make decisions or express their desires pertaining to their med-

> **Box 13–1. SPECIFIC PROVISIONS OF THE PATIENT SELF-DETERMINATION ACT**
>
> Under the act, health care facilities are currently required to do the following:
> - Ensure compliance with the requirements of state law
> - Maintain written policies and procedures with respect to advance directives
> - Provide written information to patients about their right to make decisions concerning treatment and to formulate advance directives
> - Maintain written policies and procedures with respect to advance directives
> - Document in the individual's medical record whether or not the individual has executed an advance directive
> - Educate their staff and the communities they serve about state law governing advance directives

ical treatment. Currently, some recognition of advance directives exists in all states including the District of Columbia.[3]

## Living Wills

A *living will* is much like any other will: It is a method by which wishes can be communicated when a person is unable to communicate those wishes personally. Of course, the living will deals specifically with medical treatment. Although each state has specific requirements for living wills, Figure 13–1 gives a general idea of what is included in a living will. Other specifics that may be defined by each state include the time that the living will should become effective and the limit of the treatments to which it applies.

General provisions that many states have adopted include the following:
1. The signing of the living will must be accompanied by two adult witness, one of whom must not be a spouse or blood relative.
2. Personal instructions can generally be added which allow the signer to specifically accept and refuse certain treatments, for example: "Cardiopulmonary resuscitation is acceptable, but do not use a mechanical ventilator."
3. Some states do not require living wills to be notarized.
4. A surrogate may be appointed to act on your behalf under specific conditions.

Each state also has specific instructions for revocation of living wills. Generally, revocation can be done in one of the following ways:
1. Physically destroy the original (or have someone do so for you in your presence).
2. Orally express your intent to revoke the will.
3. Write a signed and dated notice expressing your intent to revoke the will.
4. Execute a new living will that supersedes the older document.

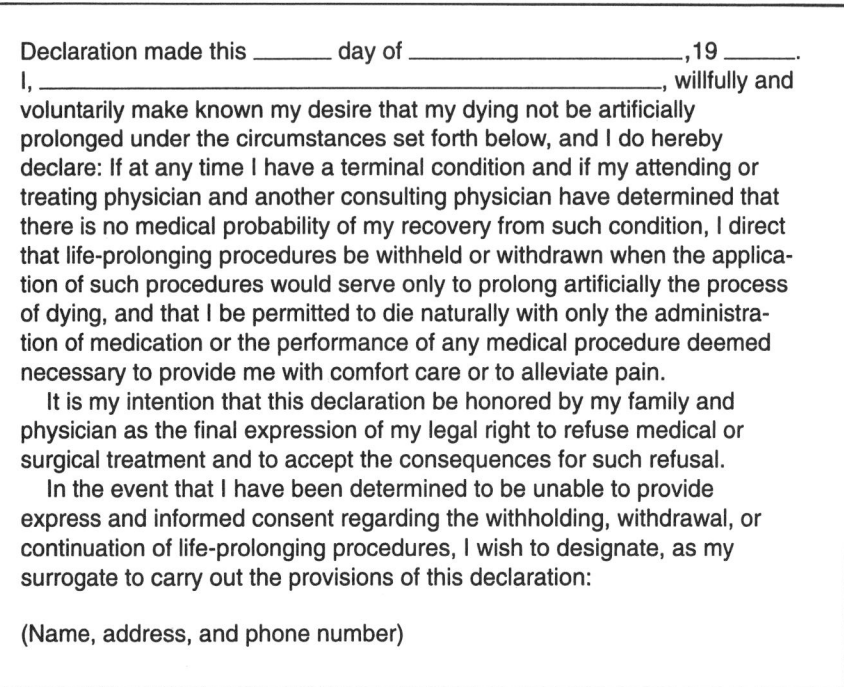

Declaration made this _____ day of _____, 19 ____.
I, _____, willfully and voluntarily make known my desire that my dying not be artificially prolonged under the circumstances set forth below, and I do hereby declare: If at any time I have a terminal condition and if my attending or treating physician and another consulting physician have determined that there is no medical probability of my recovery from such condition, I direct that life-prolonging procedures be withheld or withdrawn when the application of such procedures would serve only to prolong artificially the process of dying, and that I be permitted to die naturally with only the administration of medication or the performance of any medical procedure deemed necessary to provide me with comfort care or to alleviate pain.

It is my intention that this declaration be honored by my family and physician as the final expression of my legal right to refuse medical or surgical treatment and to accept the consequences for such refusal.

In the event that I have been determined to be unable to provide express and informed consent regarding the withholding, withdrawal, or continuation of life-prolonging procedures, I wish to designate, as my surrogate to carry out the provisions of this declaration:

(Name, address, and phone number)

**Figure 13–1.** Sample living will document

## Durable Power of Attorney for Health Care

The *durable power of attorney* differs from the living will in that rather than define specifically what steps are to be taken when one is terminally ill, it names an individual to make these decisions for the terminally ill person. Depending on the state, this appointee may be called a health care proxy, an agent, or a surrogate. Although generally the appointee (whom we will call a surrogate) acts only in end-of-life situations, in some states, the surrogate may be authorized to deal with all medical situations. Some states also allow for the appointment of an alternate surrogate. The alternate surrogate serves when the primary surrogate is unwilling or unable to serve. Probably the most important thing about the durable power of attorney is that the surrogate must clearly understand the desires of the person for whom he or she will be making decisions. Execution and revocation of the durable power of attorney for health care is very similar to the process for the living will. Figure 13–2 is a sample form for designation of the health care surrogate.

## Assisted-Suicide Activities

In mid-1990, a Detroit pathologist single-handedly began to write a new chapter in the debate on ending life. Doctor Jack Kevorkian began a movement that is now known as

> (Patient's Name)
>
> In the event that I have been determined to be incapacitated to provide informed consent for medical treatment and surgical and diagnostic procedures, I wish to designate as my surrogate for health care decisions:
>
> > (Name, address, and phone number of designee)
>
> If my surrogate is unwilling or unable to perform his duties, I wish to designate as my alternate surrogate:
>
> > (Name, address, and phone number of designee)
>
> I fully understand that this designation will permit my designee to make health care decisions and to provide, withhold, or withdraw consent on my behalf; to apply for public benefits to defray the cost of health care; and to authorize my admission to or transfer from a health care facility.
>
> > (Additional instructions if desired)
>
> I further affirm that this designation is not being made as a condition of treatment or admission to a health care facility. I will notify and send a copy of this document to the following persons other than my surrogate, so they may know who my surrogate is:
>
> (Names and addresses of those who you want to keep copies of this document)
>
> > (Signature and date of document)
>
> (Signatures and addresses of two witnesses)

**Figure 13–2.** Sample form for designation of health care surrogate

"assisted suicide." Since that time he has assisted or witnessed 21 deaths. The chapter is far from over. On April 24, 1995, the U.S. Supreme Court upheld an act passed by the State of Michigan that denounced assisted suicide, clearing the way for legal action against the pathologist who has become known in the popular press as "Dr. Death."[4]

## ETHICAL CONSIDERATIONS

The adoption of advance directives by the states, to some degree, has given answers to many of the legal questions being raised by the issue of prolonging life. When it comes to ethical considerations, however, there is still considerable debate. Although the intent of advance directives is relatively clear, there is no way in which all the situations that may arise can be anticipated. Some of the classic debate issues include questioning whether the person signing the directive was of sound mind or whether the person may have changed his or her mind based on new information since the last signing. Family members can also create complications. Very often relatives will protest the carrying out of the directive, and hospitals, afraid of legal action, find themselves in the middle of a no-win battle.

Another potential stumbling block to carrying out advance directives is the health care team itself. Ideally, there should be understanding and agreement among team members as to the proper manner in which the directives should be carried out; however, this is seldom the case. While total agreement is not required, the lack of agreement creates a problem simply because of the fear of liability if legal issues are raised concerning the carrying out of the agreement. The positive side of this entire issue is that great strides have been made toward true patient self-determination regarding medical care.

## CASE STUDY

### Case Study 13

Thomas J. is a successful businessman who works long hours. One night while driving home he becomes involved in an accident which leaves him physically in a vegetative state with his respirations supported by mechanical ventilation. Thomas had previously signed a living will in which he specifically stated he did not wish to be kept alive by artificial means. The hospital has a copy of the document. Thomas's wife, however, is hesitant to allow his wishes to be carried out. Thomas looks at her every day during visits, cries, and wonders why his wishes are not being honored.

1. What are the key legal issues?
2. What are the key ethical issues?
3. What are Thomas's rights?
4. What are his wife's rights?
5. What are the responsibilities of the health care practitioners?

## REFERENCES

1. *Cruzan v. Director,* Missouri Department of Health, U. S. Supreme Court, 88–1503.
2. Logue, B: Rights: Death Control and the Elderly in America. Macmillian, New York, 1993, p 101.
3. Hill, TP, and Shirley, D: A Good Death. Addison-Wesley, New York, 1992, pp 145–149.
4. USA Today, April 25, 1995, p 8A.

## STUDY QUESTIONS

*1. What are the essential elements of the Patient Self-Determination Act?*

2. *What are some of the complications associated with applying advance directives?*

3. *Briefly explain the difference between a living will and a durable power of attorney for health care.*

4. *Based on your previous study of ethics committees, what role do you think such a committee might be able to play in the dilemma identified in this chapter's case study?*

# CHAPTER 14

# *Allocation of Resources*

**The Issue**
Efficiency of Care
Effectiveness of Care
**Legal Considerations**
**Ethical Considerations**
**Case Study**
Case Study 14

## THE ISSUE

Although there is little agreement on appropriate solutions for resolving the crisis in available resources for health care, there is general consensus that such a crisis exists. The fact that the crisis was growing became a major issue in the 1992 presidential campaign, and it continues to challenge us today.[1] Major state and national initiatives are currently being developed to resolve the problem. Two major issues must be addressed: equal access to care for everyone and fair allocation of resources. In reality, they are not separate issues since access to care for all citizens is largely dependent on the availability of resources.

These issues are addressed primarily in the ethical principle of justice. The major dilemma incorporated within these issues is that the cost of health care is such that it is prohibitive to provide the full range of health care services to every citizen. As a point of interest, Table 14–1 contains a list of sample hospital costs from the late 1940s. It is easy to see that they do not compare exactly with current-day charges. Applied Activity 14–2 gives you the opportunity to compare the typical charges of the 1940s with current charges in your local health care facilities. "Shopping" for the

Table 14–1. TYPICAL HOSPITAL CHARGE DURING THE 1940s

| Service | Charge Per Day |
|---|---|
| Room and board | $6.75 |
| Anesthesia | 5.00 |
| Pharmacy | 1.25 |

best charge has become a reality of obtaining cost efficiency health care in today's complex health care industry.

As discussed in Chapter 3, health care costs, which were a mere $42 million in 1954, rapidly escalated to over $500 billion by 1987. The final costs for 1994 are expected to exceed a trillion dollars. How does this rapidly increasing cost compare with that of other industrialized countries? Table 14–2 gives a comparison of cost in six industrialized countries including the United States. It should be noted that although the rate of increasing cost varies considerably among countries, all the countries had extraordinary increases in the 20-year period between 1970 and 1990. And there are no indications that the rate of increase has slowed.

A factor that may impact the cost of health care is the model used to deliver care. Three basic models are currently in use in developed countries today: the national health service model, the social insurance model, and the private insurance model.[2] The national health service model provides universal coverage using a general tax-financed source of revenue. In this model, all facilities are owned by the government and all health care providers are employed by the government. This model is in use in the United Kingdom as well as in Spain, Italy, Greece, and Portugal.

The social insurance model is somewhat similar to the national health model. It is financed by contributions from both employers and employees. The system may be controlled and managed by either a governmental entity or by some other non-profit organization. Coverage is universal. The much discussed Canadian system of health care is an example of this model. France, Germany, and Japan also use variations of this model.

TABLE 14–2. COMPARISON OF SELECTED INTERNATIONAL HEALTH CARE SYSTEMS*

| Spending Per Capita | 1970 | 1990 |
|---|---|---|
| United States | $346 | $2,566 |
| Canada | 274 | 1,795 |
| France | 192 | 1,379 |
| Germany | 199 | 1,287 |
| Japan | 126 | 1,113 |
| United Kingdom | 144 | 909 |

*Source: *The Muncie Star* (Indiana), September 26, 1993.

The private insurance model is used in only two countries, the United States and South Africa. Health care facilities are privately owned and individuals either directly or through their employers purchase coverage with various defined limitations. It should be noted that in the United States, variations of both the national and social insurance models also exist. Examples include Medicaid, Medicare, the Veterans Administration, and the Public Health Service.

As current health care resources are simply not adequate to provide full care to all citizens, various forms of rationing have become a part of our health care delivery system. It should be noted, however, that there has always been some form of rationing in health care even in those cases where there has not been a deliberate effort to establish a plan or policy for rationing. The state of Oregon has taken the lead in establishing a rationing of its available Medicaid funds.[3] This was accomplished by establishing a list of priority health issues to which available funds would be applied. Due to limited funds, some items on the list of priorities will never be funded. Needless to say, the plan has created considerable controversy. Some of the realities of rationing health care are explored in Box 14–1.

Since ethical decisions are not made in a vacuum, the practical issues surrounding the allocation of resources must be explored before any reasonable ethical solutions can be considered. On a practical level, the simplest solution and the approach that would provide the most desirable ethical outcome would be to increase resources to a level that appropriate care could be provided to all citizens. Unfortunately, resources are not unlimited; therefore, this solution cannot be seriously

---

**Box 14–1.** REALITIES OF HEALTH CARE RATIONING

- *Third-Party Payers:* Almost all health care services in this country are paid for either totally or in part by some type of third-party payer. Payment is limited in various ways. Certain types of procedures or surgeries, for example, cosmetic surgery not deemed medically necessary, may not be covered. Hospital stays are also often limited.
- *Limits Imposed by Diagnosis:* Although it is logical that a patient's diagnosis would be used to determine the treatment delivered, in many cases the limits imposed by a specific diagnosis may be so restrictive that they constitute rationing.
- *Age/Prognosis:* Care provided to patients who are elderly or terminally ill are often limited to procedures that prevent suffering and provide comfort. This is to reserve resources for those patients who are better able to benefit.
- *Bureaucracy:* Third-party payers and health maintenance organizations often create a minefield of procedures that a patient must follow in order to qualify for reimbursement. The net effect is to place certain services beyond the reach of patients, resulting in a rationing of services.

considered. The next most practical solution is to look at how the current resources are being utilized, analyzing both the efficiency and effectiveness of care.

## Efficiency of Care

Efficiency of care refers to the relationship between the type of care provided and the manner in which it is provided. Theoretically, efficient care should be less expensive than inefficient care, allowing limited resources to serve a larger proportion of the population. Many who are in the midst of the debate on how to resolve the current health care crisis feel that it is the lack of an efficient health care system that is to blame for inadequate care for all citizens. Efficiency of care demands that care decisions consider the manner and cost of care as well as the outcome. The ethical principles of justice, beneficence, and nonmaleficence either directly or indirectly address the issue of efficiency of care.

As we move into the mid-1990s, upward of 35 million Americans are without any form of health insurance. The primary medical care for this growing segment of American society is provided by the various facilities that foster indigent care. Because these facilities generally cannot refuse care to these uninsured citizens, they are often filled beyond capacity. These patients seldom receive preventive or continuing care, instead they present themselves only when an acute crisis occurs. The facilities maintain that this method of providing care is inefficient and unnecessarily expensive.

## Effectiveness of Care

Effectiveness of care refers to the relationship between the care delivered and the desired outcomes. For example, if the patient is healed, even if only temporarily, the care may be deemed effective. The successful outcome, however, may not have been efficient. Effectiveness of care lends to such statements as "Do everything possible for the patient." This statement implies that cost or efficiency is less important than effectiveness. Medical technology has made and continues to make great strides. Transplants of major organs are possible. Even surgery performed on fetuses in the womb have been successful. Without question, these procedures are impressive, and they tend to give us the sense of an unlimited ability to heal and cure diseases. However, these procedures are also extremely costly, and they are seldom paid for in full by patients or their families.

## LEGAL CONSIDERATIONS

Under our current health care structure in the United States, the legal requirements associated with the allocation of resources are limited largely to those patients who receive care based on government reimbursement. Managed care contracting is also beginning to provide a systematic allocation of resources to private insurance clients. Government involvement as a payer for health care services as we know it today stems from the development of Medicaid and Medicare in the 1960s. Just as there is current opposition to plans that would provide universal coverage, the introduction of Medicaid and Medicare also met with opposition. These programs have been very successful in delivering health care to the poor and elderly; however, a major segment of our society, often termed the "working poor," is still without coverage for health care.

## ETHICAL CONSIDERATIONS

The primary ethical principle that comes to mind when the issue of allocation of resources arises is distributive justice.[4] As stated in Chapter 6, justice is easy to define but less easy to apply. Simply defined, the principle of justice would have everyone receive equal access to health care. This definition would also imply that the level of care would also be equal.

The difficulty in applying this definition is several-fold. First, comparing the delivery of health care to different individuals is like comparing applies to oranges. Individual needs differ significantly; therefore the rate and method of accessing health care also differ significantly. Furthermore, the expected outcome or prognosis differs significantly from person to person making the appropriate level of care different. In this sense, equal treatment would have to mean providing appropriate access and levels of care to each individual. The potential ethical dilemma lies in the phrase "appropriate access and levels of care."

On the face of the issue, it appears to be just and equally appropriate to provide open heart surgery to Patient A and preventive care to the pregnant mothers who make up Patients B through Z. The availability of resources, however, might make this seemingly simple comparison much more complex. What if the health care system had to choose between providing the open heart surgery *or* the prenatal care? Before attempting to answer the question posed here, a brief discussion of how patients and the health care industry might view distributive justice differently is in order. From a patient's standpoint, fair distributive justice might mean being able to access the health care system as needed while obtaining the level of care desired whenever the access is made. From the health care industry's viewpoint, fair distributive justice might mean providing the best possible care to the greatest number of individuals possible. While the patient's viewpoint is logical, it may be impossible when limited resources are considered. The health care industry's approach might be either to not perform open heart surgeries or to limit them to those patients who are most likely to benefit.

## ✓ APPLIED ACTIVITY 14–1

When considering how resources should be allocated, many opposing views tend to emerge as to who is most entitled to care. This exercise is designed to stimulate discussion of some of the more common issues. Of course, there are no absolute right or wrong answers to any of these issues. This exercise can be approached either as to an individual or as a group activity. The assignment is to rank each of the procedures according to priority in committing scarce resources.

*Situation 1*

A heart transplant for a 62-year-old recently retired worker who has been a productive tax-paying member of society or a 24-year-old college student planning to become a teacher.

*Situation 2*

A kidney transplant for a 30-year-old woman living on welfare payments with children ages 3, 5, and 7 or a 42-year-old office worker with no children.

*Situation 3*

Prenatal care program for pregnant mothers or a pulmonary rehabilitation program for emphysema patients.

##  APPLIED ACTIVITY 14-2

Determine the cost of services provided by one or more of your health care facilities. Be sure to include room cost per day, cost of anesthesia, and the costs for any selected procedures including various respiratory therapies.

## CASE STUDY

### Case Study 14

Shirley A. is a 23-year-old recently married woman with a 1-year-old child. She and her 24-year-old husband are both restaurant workers with low salaries and no health insurance benefits. Shirley is excited about being accepted into the respiratory therapy program at the local community college. She also has received approval from financial aid for her tuition and books.

The future appears to be bright with everything falling into place until Shirley takes her 1-year-old son to the local family practice clinic for what appears to be a chronic respiratory tract infection. A few weeks later, Shirley learns that her son has been diagnosed as having cystic fibrosis. Within a few months, just before classes are to start, the son's condition deteriorates rapidly. Shirley and her husband are devastated. Their immediate concern is for the health of their child; however, their concern quickly turns to the financial impact that the illness is having on the family with each passing day.

Since the family does not have health insurance, both inpatient and outpatient medical care is a major problem for the family. However, it quickly becomes obvious that their son will need extensive care at home.

The medical social worker assigned to the family informs them that home care is available but is extremely limited. Shirley quickly gives up the idea of going to school, but the problem remains—she is not skilled enough to provide all the care her son needs. The health care team members assigned to visit her son can only come once every 2 weeks due to the large number of patients needing treatment. The initial medical recommendation was that they visit twice a week. As a result of the infrequent visits, the son's medical condition continues to deteriorate.

1. What are the key legal issues?
2. What are the key ethical issues?
3. What are the responsibilities of the health care practitioners?

## STUDY QUESTIONS

1. *Some form of health care rationing has probably always been in place. What are some of the forms of rationing that you believe may have been in effect in the 1950s?*

2. *What do you see as some of the more important reasons for implementing health care rationing?*

3. *What do you see as some of the more important reasons for not implementing health care rationing?*

4. *Can you think of a situation in which you or someone you know benefited from health care rationing?*

5. *Can you think of a situation in which you or someone you know was harmed by health care rationing?*

# REFERENCES

1. Bunch, D: The health reform battle continues . . . and the clock is ticking," AARC Times, May 1994, pp 70–73.
2. *The Muncie Star* (Indiana), September 26, 1993.
3. McKenzie, JF, and Pinger, RR: An Introduction of Community Health. HarperCollins, New York, 1995, p 463.
4. Purtilo, R: Ethical Dimensions in the Health Professions, ed 2. Saunders, Philadelphia, 1993, p 205.

# CHAPTER 15

# *A Closing Perspective*

The Importance of Studying Legal Issues
 and Ethical Dilemmas
The Importance of Studying Critical
 Thinking and Systematic Decision
 Making
Understanding Word Meaning in Context
Distinguishing Between Fact and Opinion
Distinguishing Between Bias and Reason

Recognizing Deceptive Arguments
**Case Studies**
Case Study 15
Case Study 16
Case Study 17
Case Study 18
Case Study 19
Case Study 20

## THE IMPORTANCE OF STUDYING LEGAL ISSUES AND ETHICAL DILEMMAS

In addition to providing care that is technically and procedurally correct, health care practitioners must also ensure that their performance is legally and ethically correct. Today, the watchful eyes of the legal system, ethics committees, and the public as a whole maintain an ever-present vigilance over every aspect of health care delivery. As our society continues to struggle with the many issues facing health care, the environment in which practitioners work is likely to become more open to evaluation and vulnerable to accountability.

The need for an awareness and adherence to legally and ethically responsible behavior is not and should not be viewed as a burden. In fact, they should be welcomed as benchmarks of professionalism. From this standpoint, the extent to which respiratory care practitioners can demonstrate understanding and compliance with complex legal and ethical standards can be considered a measure of the advancement of the profession.

Concern for the legal rights and ethical treatment of patients is not a new issue although more and more attention is being focused on these issues as the health care system becomes increasingly complex. One of the benchmarks of concern about patient's well-being is the publishing of the document "A Patient's Bill of Rights" (see Chapter 5). The document was developed by the American Hospital Association and affirmed on February 6, 1973. It was revised in 1992. The American Hospital Association developed the "Bill of Rights" with the expectation that observance of these rights would contribute to more effective patient care and greater satisfaction for all concerned—the patient, the physician, and the hospital organization. Respiratory care practitioners, as part of the health care team, are part of the hospital organization and as such should see this document as an important guide for professional behavior and conduct.

The American Association for Respiratory Care, as the professional association for respiratory care practitioners, has also established a code of ethics that should serve as a guide for professional behavior and conduct (see Chapter 1). State respiratory care practice acts, while primarily legal documents, almost always deal with the ethical dilemmas related to professional practice. The efforts by these varied groups should impress upon both the new and the experienced respiratory care practitioner the importance of legal and ethical issues in the practice of respiratory care.

Of course, no document can ensure that patients will receive the kind of treatment they desire. Furthermore, no document can predict all the unique situations that combine to create legal issues and ethical dilemmas that are likely to arise during the delivery of care; however, these documents are major steps in the right direction. The ethical principles, theories, and decision-making models presented in this book are a continuation of the efforts initiated by these documents. It is the responsibility of the serious and committed practitioner to continue to consider the legal and ethical dilemmas associated with the practice of respiratory care. That commitment is not only important for the advancement of patient care, it is also important for the profession.

## THE IMPORTANCE OF STUDYING CRITICAL THINKING AND SYSTEMATIC DECISION MAKING

The ability to think critically is essential if health care professionals are to be able to resolve ethical dilemmas effectively. At this point, after many discussions of ethical and legal dilemmas, exploration of decision-making models, and case study analysis, the reality is that without the ability to think critically, the practitioner will be unable to objectively apply the information learned up to this point. To teach ethics without also teaching critical thinking leads to indoctrination rather than ethical insight.[1]

This overview of critical thinking skills will cover four areas that health care professionals need to be constantly aware of as they deal with ethical dilemmas[2,3]:
- Understanding word meaning in context
- Distinguishing between fact and opinion

- Distinguishing bias from reason
- Recognizing deceptive arguments

## Understanding Word Meaning in Context

Most words have several meanings, with the exact meaning depending on the context in which they are used. When both familiar and unfamiliar key words are encountered, it is important that an effort be made to determine their meaning in the specific situation. This can often be done by carefully reading the statement containing the word, looking up the word in a dictionary, and reading the surrounding statements. The most important thing, however, is to be aware that word meaning does vary when the context changes. A classic term used in respiratory care is "respiratory distress." Every respiratory care practitioner recognizes the term and will immediately formulate a meaning when it is used to describe a patient's condition. In reality, however, unless objective data are included with the term, the meaning attached to the term will vary widely between individuals. Such terms as "quality of life" and "maximum care" can be as easily confused.

## Distinguishing Between Fact and Opinion

Any discussion of controversial issues is likely to contain numerous statements of both fact and opinion. It is important to recognize each type of statement and to realize that not all statements of "fact" are true since they may be based on inaccurate data. Statements of fact may have a measurable or quantitative component. Such statements may also be simply a statement that appears to be true, and the reader or listener cannot contradict it without further information. Statements of opinion tend to be qualitative rather than quantitative. While it is not always easy to distinguish between these two types of statements, it is extremely important to try. In order to distinguish between fact and opinion effectively, one must be willing not only to question statements on the surface but also to question the underpinnings of the statement. A simple statement such as "Patient A always refuses his treatment and wants to die" sounds straightforward on the surface. In reality, it is possible that the patient has refused some treatments but has no desire to die. The first part of the statement could be a fact, although the word "always" significantly decreases the likelihood that it is. The second part could also be a fact if this information has been clearly communicated by the patient. However, if the second part of the statement is based on the first part, it can only be an opinion and a dangerous conclusion of the speaker.

## Distinguishing Between Bias and Reason

When discussing highly controversial issues, there is a tendency by many people to allow their emotions to dominate their normal rational reasoning. Thus, the ability to distinguish between bias and reason is extremely important for the health care professional attempting to resolve ethical dilemmas. Again, this is not always easy to do. In attempting to make the distinction, it should be remembered that statements of reason will generally be fact-based and will have a logical flow based on a series of rational deductions. Statements of bias will generally not be fact-based.

Facts, if present, however, may be distorted in order to conform to a bias. Suppose, for example, that a male patient is admitted to the hospital and remains for several weeks. The only person ever to visit this patient is another man who always embraces the patient and with whom the patient always talks in quiet, almost secretive, tones. A staff member who dislikes homosexuals starts a rumor that the man is the patient's lover. It is later learned that the patient's diagnosis is Pneumocystis carinii pneumonia, an opportunistic disease associated with acquired immunodeficiency syndrome. In the minds of many staff members, the diagnosis confirms the patient's homosexuality and the visiting lover rumor. In fact, the visitor is a business partner who is arranging to care for the patient's family. Furthermore, the patient is not a homosexual; he contracted the human immunodeficiency virus from a blood transfusion.

## Recognizing Deceptive Arguments

Deceptive arguments are designed to distract listeners or readers from the real issues and persuade them to agree with the person advancing the argument. Such arguments may appeal to the emotions or even to the intellect of the individuals to whom they are addressed. Again, it is extremely important to be able to recognize deceptive arguments, but not always easy to do so. Some of the appeals commonly utilized are listed below:

1. *Groupthink or bandwagon.* The idea in this technique is to convince the listener or reader that this "fact" is believed by everyone. Be aware of statements that begin with "*Everyone* knows that . . ." or "*All* those people . . ."
2. *Personal attacks.* This technique focuses on engaging in personal attacks on anyone who disagrees with the belief of the person advancing the argument. Watch for statements such as "If you were *smart*, you would understand . . ." or "What do you *expect* from someone like that?"
3. *Testimonial.* In this instance, an authority figure or celebrity is quoted to prove support for a specific viewpoint. The testimonial is commonly invoked in health care facilities with statements such as "Dr. Smith ways it's true" or "Dr. Smith agrees with me." Note that it is important to respect authority figures but that if the authority is valid, it can withstand the scrutiny of questions.
4. *Generalizations.* This technique used an isolated fact for an individual and applies it to entire populations. It is similar to saying that what is true for "a" is also true for "b" through "z" simply because they are all letters of the alphabet.

There are numerous "tricks" used in deceptive arguments. Careful listening and critical thinking and systematic decision making will assist in recognizing most of these invalid arguments. The analysis, or problem-solving, method of ethical decision making presented in Chapter 6 is an excellent tool for systematic decision making.

**154** Applications and Practices

## ✓ CAPSTONE ACTIVITY

This final activity is designed both to increase the learner's awareness of current ethical issues and to provide the learner with another opportunity to engage in applied ethical decision making. The assignment is as follows: During the next month, note any stories in your local newspaper dealing with health care issues that may have ethical implications. Document your reaction to the stories prior to discussing the issues involved with anyone else. Then discuss the issues with two to three other people and document their reactions. Compare the reactions noting how they have been affected by other personal or societal events that may be occurring. Attempt to develop your critical thinking skills as you carry out this activity. Utilized to its fullest, this activity will assist you in refining your skills in dealing with dilemmas. Good luck!

## CASE STUDIES

### Case Study 15

Tina R. is registered respiratory therapist in a 350-bed for-profit hospital. She is participating in a clinical conference concerning the appropriate care for a premature infant who has moderate respiratory distress. The conference participants all agree that it would be wise to place the infant on a ventilator immediately to decrease the chance of brain damage. Tina points out that all of the department's respirators are in use on more critical patients. Efforts to rent an additional respirator immediately have been unsuccessful. The rental company has indicated that it would be at least 24 hours before they would be able to deliver a respirator. The pediatric resident points out that one of the critical patients using a respirator has an extremely poor prognosis and already appears to be brain dead. She suggests that this patient be "weaned" in order to free the respirator. She reasons that the infant with the moderate distress has an excellent chance of surviving and having a healthy life if she is placed on the respirator immediately. However, without it, she is likely to have brain damage. The other infant will die anyway, she states emphatically.

1. What are the key legal issues?
2. What are the key ethical issues?
3. Who has rights in this case and what are they?
4. What are the responsibilities of the health care practitioners?

### Case Study 16

Joel W. is a reformed smoker who now has an adamant antismoker attitude. He lectures all of his patients on the importance of not smoking. As a pulmonary rehabilitation therapist, his lectures are sometimes appropriate. In addition to working in the rehabilitation program during the week, Joel sometimes works in the respiratory care department on weekends.

One Saturday afternoon, Joel is called to the emergency room to assist a patient who has just come in with severe respiratory distress. Upon entering the emergency room, Joel recognizes the patient as Mr. Norman, one of his pulmonary rehabilitation patients. Mr. Norman has a strong smell of smoke on his breath and clothes. As Joel is setting up oxygen for the patient, he asks Mr. Norman if he has been smoking. Mr. Norman states that he has and that his smoking doesn't matter since he's going to die soon anyway. Joel becomes angry and immediately begins to lecture Mr. Norman loudly. Mr. Norman, who is already noticeably in distress, becomes even more distressed. His heart rate begins to increase immediately, and within a few minutes he is in ventricular tachycardia.

1. What are the key legal issues?
2. What are the key ethical issues?
3. Did Joel have a right to lecture this patient about smoking while the patient is attending rehabilitation classes? while the patient is the emergency room?

## Case Study 17

Shirley P. is the evening shift supervisor in a large metropolitan hospital. As part of her duties, she becomes familiar with Mr. Johnson, a long-term ventilator patient with a terminal prognosis. He has been on the ventilator for 5 months with no chance of weaning or recovering. The patient's family decides to take Mr. Johnson home for his final days. Several therapists, including Shirley, are employed to assist in Mr. Johnson's home care. Shirley agrees to work the night shift at Mr. Johnson's home immediately following her hospital shift. On her first night at Mr. Johnson's home she is greeted by Mr. Johnson's son who tells her to sit in the family room and relax for a moment. Shirley does so and promptly falls asleep. She awakens about 20 minutes later and attempts to enter the room where Mr. Johnson is on the ventilator. The door is locked. She knocks. The son opens the door, and immediately Shirley notices that the ventilator has been turned off. The son advised Shirley that his father had died a few minutes earlier. Shirley feels extremely uncomfortable. She wonders if she has been negligent, and if the son somehow took part in Mr. Johnson's death.

1. What are the key legal issues?
2. What are the key ethical issues?
3. What are Shirley's responsibilities?
4. Should she share with anyone her suspicions about the son?

## Case Study 18

Tom R. is a 40-year-old registered therapist working the evening shift in a small private hospital. One of the marketing tools of the hospital is that it provides a homelike environment for its patients. All patients have private rooms, wear their personal sleepwear, and enjoy wine with their dinner, unless it is medically prohibited. One of Tom's patients is a 38-year-old very attractive woman, Tammy C., who seems to have developed an attraction for Tom. She is receiving aerosol therapy for asthma. For 3 days in a row, during her last treatment she has insisted that Tom drink a glass of wine that she has set aside for him from her dinner. Tom refuses the first day; however, he gives in and drinks the wine the following 2 days. He reasons that he is just being friendly and that one glass of wine will not be a problem. On the fourth night when Tom enters the room, the patient asks to close the door and again offers him a glass of wine. Tom drinks the wine. The patient tells Tom that she is going home the following day and that she would like to see him after her discharge. She writes her phone number on a piece of paper and hands it to Tom. She then asks Tom to hug her.

1. Should Tom hug this patient?
2. Should Tom have drunk the wine offered by the patient?
3. What are the key ethical issues?
4. Should Tom call his patient after her discharge?
5. What are the responsibilities of health care practitioners in regard to personal relationships with patients?

## Case Study 19

Jenny A. is a registered respiratory therapist employed by a new and struggling home care company. As part of her employment package, Jenny is told that she will receive bonuses if the company performs well. Jenny is unfamiliar with the third-party reimbursement procedures for home care. Her boss, who is also the company owner, assures her that he will assist her with the charting to ensure that the company receives the best possible reimbursement. This arrangement continues for several months, and Jenny earns several bonus checks since the company is performing well. Jenny assumes everything is fine until she attends a workshop on Medicare fraud. The workshop leaves Jenny curious about the manner in which she is charting certain patient information. She decides to review some of her previous charting, and to her astonishment she realizes that she has been involved in Medicare fraud. She suspects that her boss has known this all along.

1. What are the key legal issues?
2. What are the key ethical issues?
3. What should Jenny do at this point?

## Case Study 20

Ashleigh O. is a registered respiratory therapist working in a small hospital in a large city. While checking a patient's chart, she discovers information that leads her to the conclusion that the patient is HIV-positive. She thinks very little about the information until she receives a phone call from a friend the following day. The friend tells her that the patient is a former boyfriend of hers and asks how he is doing.

1. What are the key legal issues?
2. What are the key ethical issues?
3. What should Ashleigh tell her friend?

## REFERENCES

1. Paul, R: Critical Thinking: What Every Person Needs to Survive in a Rapidly Changing World. The Foundation for Critical Thinking, Santa Rosa, CA, 1992, p 240.
2. Flight, MR: Law, Liability and Ethics. Delmar, Albany, NY, 1988.
3. Bach, JS (Ed): Biomedical Ethics: Opposing Viewpoints. Greenhaven Press, St. Paul, MN, 1987.

# Index

AARC. *See* American Association of Respiratory Care
Abortion, 7
Acquired immunodeficiency syndrome (AIDS), 114, 115, 118
Advance directives, 133–141
 assisted-suicide activities, 138–139
 case study 13, 140
 durable power of attorney for health care, 138, 139
 ethical considerations, 139–140
 legal considerations, 136–139
 living wills, 137, 138
 ordinary vs. extraordinary care, 135–136
 in patient's bill of rights, 64
Advocacy, 43
AIDS (acquired immunodeficiency syndrome), 114, 115, 118
Allocation of resources, 35, 142–149
 case study 14, 147–148
 effectiveness of care and, 145
 efficiency of care and, 145
 ethical considerations, 146
 health insurance models and, 143–144
 legal considerations, 145–146
American Association of Respiratory Care (AARC)
 code of ethics, 8, 151
 and licensure, 21
American Health Information Management Association, 92
American legal system, 12–18. *See also* Laws
 courts and the trial process, 17–18
 sources and types of laws, 13–17
American Medical Association Judicial Council, 44
Analysis method, 74–77
 case studies, 83, 84–86, 87
Assault and battery, 25
Assisted-suicide, 138–139
Attitudes, personal, 31
Attitudinal orientation, 31
Autonomy, 43–44, 52, 53, 57, 86
 deontological theory and, 71
 human experimentation and, 102
Autopsy, 93

Bankowski, Zbigniew, 43
Battery, 25
Beliefs, personal, 31
Beneficence, 52, 53, 57
 deontological theory and, 71
 human experimentation and, 102
Bentham, Jeremy, 72
Bias vs. reason, 152–153
Bill of rights, patient's, 62, 63–66, 90, 151
Bioethics, 31
Brain death, 125. *See also* Dying patients
 case study 12, 130
 guidelines for determining, 127
Burden of proof, 16

Centers for Disease Control, 15
Certification
 defined, 20–21
 national, 19–21
Certified Respiratory Therapy Technician (CRTT), 19
Child abuse, need to report, 93
Chronic illness, 113, 114. *See also* Terminally ill
 case study 10, 117
 guidelines for delivery of care, 115
 legal considerations, 115
Chronic obstructive pulmonary disease (COPD), 114, 116
Civil law, 13, 15–16
 trials, 18
Columbia University, 5
Coma, irreversible, 125
Common law, English, 12, 13
Common practice, experimental care vs., 99
Communicable diseases, 113, 114–115
 case study 11, 118
 ethical considerations, 115–116
 guidelines for delivery of care, 116–117
 legal considerations, 115
 need to report, 91, 93
Conditions of Participation for Hospitals in Medicare and Medical Programs, 93
Conditions of Participation for Long-Term Care Facilities, 93

Confidentiality, 7, 34, 90–97
  appropriate times to break, 91
  case studies, 95–96
  deontological theory and, 72
  ethical considerations, 95
  as ethical principle, 52, 53–54, 57
  issue of, 90–92
  legal considerations, 92–95
  material covered by, 91, 92
  in patient's bill of rights, 64
Consent, patient's
  informed, 101. *See also* Informed consent
  in research and human experimentation, 64
Constitution
  state, 14
  U.S., 13–14
Continuity of care, patient's right to, 65
Court system, 17–18
Credentialing, legal, 9
Criminal law, 13, 15, 17
  trials, 18
Critically ill, guidelines for care, 122–123
Critical thinking, 151–153
  case studies, 154–157
CRTT (Certified Respiratory Therapy Technician), 19

Dartmouth College, 5
Death, brain, 125. *See also* Dying patients
  case study 12, 130
  guidelines for determining, 127
Death protocols, 127–128
Deceptive arguments, 153
Decision making
  ethical. *See* Ethical decision making
  importance of systematic, 151–153
  patient participation in, 46, 65, 109
Defamation, 25
Delivery of care, guidelines for, 116–117
Demanding extraordinary attention (patients), 107
Deontological theory, 33, 69–72
  case study, 81–82
Difficult patients, 105–112
  case study, 111
  defining, 105–106
  demanding extraordinary attention, 107
  ethical considerations, 110
  legal considerations, 109
  noncompliance, 106, 107
  patient-centered care and, 109
  rules for dealing with, 110
  therapeutic communication, 110–111
  "undesirables," 108
  violating hospital rules, 107–108
Disclosure, informed consent and, 101
Disease care, health care vs., 37–38
Diseases, ethics and, 33–36
Do Not Resuscitate (DNR) orders, 34, 126

Durable power of attorney for health care, 138, 139
Dying patients, 124–126. *See also* Terminally ill patients
  ethical considerations, 128–130
  legal considerations, 126–127

Effectiveness of care, allocation of resources and, 145
Efficiency of care, allocation of resources and, 145
Electroencephalogram (EEG), and brain death, 125–126
Empirical evidence, 47
Empirical statements, 47–48
English common law, 12, 13
Entitlement to health care, 36–37
Equal treatment (justice) for patients, 35
Equitable relief, 16
Ethical autonomy, 43–44
Ethical considerations
  advance directives, 139–140
  allocation of resources, 146
  chronic illness and communicable disease, 115–116
  confidentiality, 95
  difficult patients, 110
  human experimentation, 102
  importance of, 150–151
  for respiratory care practitioners, 9–10
  terminally ill and dying patients, 128–130
Ethical decision making, 41–50, 151
  applied, 79–89. *See also specific case studies*
  basis of, 41–42
  individual process, 46–47
  participating in, 44–48
  as process, 45–46
  responsibility for, 42–44
Ethical guidelines, 13
Ethical issues. *See also* Ethical considerations *and specific case studies*
  history of, 5–8
Ethical orientation, 31
Ethical principles (standards), 32–33, 46, 51–67, 151
  autonomy, 52, 53, 57
  beneficence, 52, 53, 57
  confidentiality, 52, 53–54, 57, 95. *See also* Confidentiality
  fidelity, 52, 54, 57
  justice, 52, 54, 57
  nonmaleficence, 52, 54, 57
  paternalism, 52, 57, 62
  patient's bill of rights, 62, 63–66
  quality of life, 52, 57–58, 62
  reparation, 52, 58, 62
  sanctity of life, 52, 58–59, 62
  traditional vs. contemporary, 51–62
  utilitarianism, 52, 59, 62
  veracity, 52, 59–60, 62

Ethical theories, 33, 46, 68–78, 151
  analysis method, 74–77
  deontological, 33, 69–72
  utilitarian, 33, 72–74
Ethical thinking, foundation of, 31–33
Ethics
  bio-, 31
  definitions of, 30–31
  evolution of professional codes of, 6–8
  health, disease and, 33–36
  and health care, 30–40, 38
  and laws, 14
  nonnormative, 31
  normative, 31
  professional, 31
    evolution of codes, 6–8
Ethics committees, 44–45
Euthanasia, 7
Evaluative statements, 47–48
Experimental care. *See also* Human experimentation
  common practice vs., 99
Extended care facilities, guidelines for care in, 123–124
Extraordinary vs. ordinary care, 135–136

Fact vs. opinion, 152
Federal laws, 13–17. *See also* Laws
Felonies, 17
Fidelity, 52, 54, 57, 86, 116
Food and Drug Administration, 15
Formalist theory. *See* Deontological theory

Generalizations, 153
German concentration camps, 98, 100
Gilligan, Carol, 32, 42
"Greater weight of evidence," 16
Groupthink, 153

Health, Education, and Welfare, Department of, guidelines on human experimentation, 101
Health care
  disease care vs., 37–38
  as entitlement, 36–37
  extraordinary vs. ordinary, 135–136
  role of ethics in, 38
Health care costs, 143
Health care delivery models, 143–144
Health care proxy, 138
Health care rationing, 144
Hepatitis B, 114, 115
Hippocratic oath, 6–8, 90
HIV (human immunodeficiency virus), 114, 115
Hospice care, 122–123
Hospital policies, patient's right to know, 65

Human experimentation, 98–104
  common practice vs. experimental care, 99
  ethical considerations, 102
  HEW guidelines on, 101
  legal considerations, 101–102
  patient's consent to, 64, 101
Human immunodeficiency virus (HIV), 114, 115

Impaired performance, professional, 35
Incompetence, professional, 35
Informed consent, 101
  components of doctrine, 129
  and terminal illness, 129
Insurance, health, models of, 143–144
Insurance, liability, 27
  evolution of, 6
Intentional tort, 24–25
Invasion of privacy, 25

Joint Committee on Accreditation of Healthcare Organizations (JCAHO), 27, 44
Justice, 52, 54, 57
  and allocation of resources, 142, 146

Kant, Immanuel, 33, 69
Kevorkian, Dr. Jack, 138–139
Kohlberg, Lawrence, 32, 42

Laws
  civil, 13, 15–16
  criminal, 13, 15, 17
  ethics and, 14
  societal values and, 14
  sources and types of, 13–17
  state, 15
Legal basis for respiratory care practice, 18–24
  national registration and certification, 19–21
  state acts, 21–24
Legal considerations
  advance directives, 136–139
  allocation of resources, 145–146
  chronic illness and communicable disease, 115
  confidentiality, 92–95
  difficult patients, 109
  human experimentation, 101–102
  importance of, 150–151
  terminally ill and dying patients, 126–127
Legal credentialing. *See* Credentialing, legal
Legal issues. *See also* Legal considerations
  case study, 9
  history of, 5–8
  for respiratory care practitioners, 9
Legal scope of practice, 43–44

Legal system, American, 12–18
  courts and the trial process, 17–18
  sources and types of laws, 13–17
Level of care, 107
Liability in respiratory care practice, 24–27
  malpractice prevention, 26–27
  malpractice protection, 27
  professional, 24–26
Liability insurance, 27
  evolution of, 6
Libel, 25
Licensing, 9–10
Licensing eligibility, 23–24
Licensing fees, 24
Licensing laws, state, 20
Licensing process, 24
Licensure. *See also* Respiratory Care Practice Acts
  defined, 20
  function of, 21
  states with, 23
Life support, termination of, 34
Life support equipment, and the dying patient, 124–125
Listening, active and reflective, 111
Living wills, 137, 138

Malpractice
  evolution of, 6
  prevention, 26–27
  professional, tort law and, 26
  protection, 27
Medicaid, 144, 146
Medical ethicist, 45
Medical ethics. *See* Ethics
Medical training, history of, 5–6
Medicare, 144, 146
  cost of, 37
Mill, John Stuart, 33, 72
Minors, decision making for, 43
Misdemeanors, 17
*Missouri v. Cruzan*, 136
Monetary damages, 16
Moral development, Kohlberg on, 32
Moral orientation, 32
Morals, personal, 31

Napoleonic code, 13
National Board for Respiratory Care (NBRC), 19
National health service model, 143
National Hospice Organization, 123
National Institutes of Health, 15
National registration and certification, 19–21
Nazi concentration camps, 98, 100
Negligence, tort law and, 25–26
Noncompliant patients, 106, 107
Nonmaleficence, 52, 54, 57, 116
  human experimentation and, 102
Nonnormative ethics, 31

Normative ethics, 31
Nuremberg Code, 100–101

Opinion vs. fact, 152
Order forms, 18
Ordinary vs. extraordinary care, 135–136
Organ transplantation, 126–127

Parent–minor relationship, 43
Paternalism, 52, 57, 62
  deontological theory and, 71
Patient(s)
  and decision making, 46, 65, 109
  difficult, 105–112. *See also* Difficult patients
  responsibility for providing information, 65
Patient-centered care, 109
Patient confidentiality. *See* Confidentiality
Patient-family conflict, 35
Patient's bill of rights, 62, 63–66, 90, 151
Patient Self-Determination Act, 136, 137
Patient's right to know
  and hospital policies, 65
  and terminal illness, 128–129
Pay for services, inability of patient to, 35
Pennsylvania Hospital, 5
Permission form (patient). *See also* Consent
  failure to obtain, 25
Personal attacks, 153
Personal attitudes, 31
Personal beliefs, 31
Personal morals, 31
Personal values, 31–32
Plaintiff, 16
Preventive care, 37
Privacy. *See also* Confidentiality
  invasion of, 25
  in patient's bill of rights, 64, 92
Privacy Act of 1974, 93
Private insurance model, 143, 144
Problem-solving method. *See* Analysis method
Professional ethics, 31
  evolution of codes of, 6–8
Professionalism, 19
  defined by Public Law 93-360, 20
Professional liability, 24–26
Professional malpractice, tort law and, 26
Prosecuting attorney, 17
Public health reporting, 91, 93
Public Law 93-360, 19, 20
Public Reporting Statutes, 95

Quality assurance, 27
Quality of care, 107
Quality of life, 52, 57–58, 62
  and advance directives, 134
  defining, 134
Quinlan case, 44

Reason vs. bias, 152–153
Records
  computerization of, 92
  confidentiality of, 91. See also Confidentiality
  falsification of, 17
  patient's right to review, 64
Reflexes, brain death and, 125
Registered Nurse, 20
Registered Respiratory Therapist (RRT), 19
Registration
  defined, 20, 21
  national, 19–21
Regulatory agencies, 14
Research, patient's consent to, 64
Res ipsa loquitur, 26
Resource allocation. See Allocation of resources
Respiratory care practice
  experimental care in, 99
  legal basis for, 18–24
    national registration and certification, 19–21
    state acts, 21–24
  liability in
    malpractice prevention, 26–27
    malpractice protection, 27
    professional, 24–26
Respiratory Care Practice Acts, 15. See also Licensure
  components of, 22–24
  states with, 23
Respondeat superior, 19
Restitution, 12–13
Risk management, 27
  evolution of, 6

Sanctity of life, 52, 58–59, 62
  deontological theory and, 71
Slander, 25
Social insurance model, 143
Societal values, laws and, 14
Staffing, inadequate, 35
Standard of care, 26–27
State acts on respiratory care practice, 21–24
State constitutions, 14
State courts, 17–18
State laws, 15. See also Laws
Step-by-step analysis. See Analysis method
Suicide, assisted, 138–139
Surrogate, 138

Terminally ill patients, 121, 122–124. See also Dying patients
  ethical considerations, 128–130
  guidelines for care, 122, 123–124
  legal considerations, 126–127
Termination of life support, 34
Testimonials, 153
Therapeutic communication, 110–111
Title protection
  defined, 21
  states with, 21, 22
Tort law, 24–26
  intentional, 24–25
  negligence, 25–26
Trial process, 17–18
  by jury, 16
Tuberculosis, drug-resistant, 114
Tuskegee Institute experiments, 99

"Undesirables," 108
Uniform Brain Death Act, 126
Uniform Death Act, 127
Uniform Health Care Information Act, 93
Utilitarianism, 52, 59, 62
Utilitarian theory, 33, 72–74
  case study, 82–83

Values
  personal, 31–32
  societal, 14
Veracity, 52, 59–60, 62
Violation of hospital rules by patients, 107–108

Word meaning in context, 152

ISBN 0-8036-0126-3